AFRICAN AMERICAN
HERBALISM

AFRICAN AMERICAN
HERBALISM

A Practical Guide to Healing Plants
and Folk Traditions

Lucretia VanDyke

Published by:
ULYSSES PRESS
PO Box 3440
Berkeley, CA 94703
www.ulyssespress.com

ISBN: 978-1-64604-352-1
Library of Congress Control Number: 2022932778

Printed in the United States by Versa Press
10 9 8 7 6 5 4 3 2

Acquisitions editor: Kierra Sondereker
Managing editor: Claire Chun
Editor: Michele Anderson
Proofreader: Renee Rutledge
Interior design and layout: Winnie Liu
Illustrations and cover art: Catherine McElvane

NOTE TO READERS: This book has been written and published strictly for informational and educational purposes only. It is not intended to serve as medical advice or to be any form of medical treatment. You should always consult your physician before altering or changing any aspect of your medical treatment and/or undertaking a diet regimen. Do not stop or change any prescription medications without the guidance and advice of your physician. Any use of the information in this book is made on the reader's good judgment after consulting with his or her physician and is the reader's sole responsibility. This book is not intended to diagnose or treat any medical condition and is not a substitute for a physician.

This book is independently authored and published and no sponsorship or endorsement of this book by, and no affiliation with, any trademarked brands or other products mentioned within is claimed or suggested. All trademarks that appear in ingredient lists and elsewhere in this book belong to their respective owners and are used here for informational purposes only. The author and publisher encourage readers to patronize the brands mentioned in this book.

I dedicate these pages first and foremost to the ancestors both known and unknown. To the plants, which have always been my friends, and to all of you, my fellow herbalists and herbal enthusiasts. May these words help you on your own healing journey and inspire you to be storytellers, be keepers of your traditions, be there for your community, and "work the roots" with love.

CONTENTS

CHAPTER 4 SPIRITUAL BATHING WITH THE ELEMENTS

INTRODUCTION

My journey as an herbalist has taken me to many faraway exotic lands, but the work in my own land has been the most life changing.

During my studies in the US, I heard people sing songs to the plants and listened to stories about herbalism. While these stories were helpful, they did not fully represent people of color. They did not resonate as deeply until I began the journey to find my own people's story—that of African Americans and other people of African descent—with these plants. Many times I would hear my teachers speak about a person of color who influenced their path to herbalism, but their names were long forgotten. Who were these herbalists who were lost to history?

But first, let me explain what herbal medicine, or herbalism, is. Herbal medicine has a long history, with a written history dating back more than five thousand years, according to the American Herbalists Guild. "Herbal medicine is the art and science of using plants to support health and wellness. Herbalists are people who dedicate their lives to working with medicinal plants. Many have an intimate relationship with plants and their medicinal value."[1] Often referred to as phytotherapy or botanical medicine, herbal medicine is one of the earliest systems of medicine known to humankind.

---

1 "Herbal Medicine FAQs," American Herbalists Guild, accessed October 15, 2021, https://www.americanherbalistsguild.com/herbal-medicine-fundamentals.

In my travels, in what I learned from indigenous healers, and in my studies of my own culture, I have found that herbalism is a practice steeped in the traditions of reverence for the human connection to mother earth and her vast resources for healing the body, mind, and soul. Herbalism addresses both the physical and spiritual aspects of plants. Herbal practitioners have a deep and multilayered understanding of how plants are used as medicines. Furthermore, in their holistic approach to healing and their use of plants in spiritual ceremonies, herbalists are also attuned—on so many levels—to the connection of plants to the spiritual world.

Herbal medicine differs from much of modern conventional medicine, which is based on scientific evidence and is designed to treat physical symptoms and diseases through medications or invasive methods.[2] Instead, herbal medicine focuses on a person's participation in their own health and wellness through diet and physical and mental exercise, as well as the use of the medicines of the earth, such as the roots of burdock or poke, pine needles, and onions. We herbalists belong to a culture in which we followed the ways taught to our ancestors of Africa and the Caribbean, and we used what we learned from the Native people of this land. We weaved these practices together here in the United States and created our own folk traditions from those passed down to us by our grandmothers' grandmothers through oral tradition.

When I was researching the herbalism of the American South, I came across a book written about native Southern plants. Its author had written about the "research of the remedies," including old tales of how using the saliva of highly melanated people—that is, Black people—was said to cure things that "ailed" you, as well as how using children as footstools cured rheumatoid arthritis. Yes, folk medicine stories do exist, but what the author wrote afterward was shocking. He said

---

2 Lisa A. Kisling, Regan A. Stiegmann, "Alternative Medicine," https://pubmed.ncbi.nlm.nih.gov/30860755, July 26, 2021.

that he believed that enslaved people were "taking advantage of people who were white."[3] Really, he said this—unbelievable! I was thinking to myself, "This cannot be our only story." That moment of realization inspired my lecture about walking in the legacy of healers of color and ultimately led to my writing this book.

As my curiosity took hold, I began a quest to collect the stories of these healers, to find out who we of African descent were before we got to America, and to speak the names of the women and cultures that were so important to preserving the old ways—these powerful people who wove a patchwork quilt of knowledge passed down from those ancestral lands that most their descendants have forgotten or never felt the sunrise in.

There is no way to fully know about all the accomplishments and contributions of people of color in the healing arts, just like our history cannot be told in a single month. I can speak the names of only a few people and countries that have influenced me as a healer, medicine woman, and herbalist. I have used their stories as a guide and inspiration when creating plant medicine, and doing so has made me a better herbalist as well as a better person.

I have been lecturing about our Black history of herbalism and the healing arts for over a decade. I do this to inspire each of us to use these plants as they were intended—to heal—and to encourage us to turn toward each other as a community.

Elders in many circles I have joined have told stories, passed down as part of oral tradition, about how people of African descent—our people—have always been travelers.[4] Sadly, untold numbers of our ancestors were also taken away from their homes in Africa to be enslaved in the

---

3 Anthony Cavender, *Folk Medicine in Southern Appalachia* (Chapel Hill: University of North Carolina Press, 2003), 51–53.
4 *The History and Legacy of the 1619 Enslaved African Landing*, directed by Calvin Pearson (Project 1619 Inc., 2021).

Americas with nothing but their prayers to the ancestors and their fear of the unknown in their hearts. Our ancestors did, however, take with them the knowledge that they would need the native medicines wherever they were taken to. They would combine the medicines from different shores, from their ancestral homes, with the knowledge from ancient times.

These plant medicines and methodologies spread from generation to generation, handed down from grandmothers, mothers, and aunties through stories, songs, and practical use of the herbs, intertwined with the knowledge of the importance of the plants' connection to the earth. I believe that when you have a deep connection to these plants, they will tell you how they are medicine if you let them. These chapters are meant to inspire through storytelling and, as we say, "working the roots" to create plant medicine to help heal the mind, body, and soul.

These chapters are also meant to remind people of African descent of who we were before we came to the Americas and of the deep legacy that is ours. Each page is meant to inspire each of you to dive deep into your own ancestral connection to these plants and honor those whose DNA is in you. Without this knowledge of plant medicine being passed down, none of us would be here today. I am truly excited and honored to share these stories and recipes with you.

So grab a cup of tea and let me take you on a journey from ancient Egypt ... to other areas of Africa ... through the Middle Passage ... to America and straight to my homeland in the southern Appalachian Mountains.

CHAPTER 1

THE HISTORY OF AFRICAN AMERICAN HERBALISM

Ancient Egypt

Many philosophies of medicine have inspired African American herbalism, and I cannot address them all in this book. I can speak only of the ones that have influenced my path as a medicine woman and my personal journey of understanding the healing arts and our connection to plants. Most important, I believe we must know more about where we come from and who we are to help us reclaim our narratives.

Thinking about how far back our history in the healing arts goes, I have always been inspired by ancient Egypt. Many narratives about medicine cite the Greeks as being extremely influential. In my research, however, I have found that while the ancient Egyptians and those in the surrounding areas on the African continent have significantly influenced the medical paths to health and wellness, they are often not as recognized as the Greeks in modern times. The spread of this influence was made accessible by the Nile River, on which explorers took this knowledge and spread it far and wide for others to incorporate and be inspired by, and ultimately—and very much later in history—the Middle Passage (a transatlantic slave trade route). The ancient civilizations of Egypt and other parts of Africa established a foundation for medicine, writing down and documenting their finds.

Like our ancestors from this continent, we as a people are deeply connected to how the human body works. With the right environment, diet, plant medicine, close attention to the spiritual side of healing, and communion with nature, we can bring physical and spiritual balance back to ourselves. I see how greatly the past has influenced us in ways we may not even know, and how we keep adapting the past to the times. The past is a part of our story and our legacy that we carry with us in our bones, as you will see in these pages.

Sound as a Healing Force

Many of the practices of modern herbal medicine, such as using sound as an agent of healing, originate in ancient Egypt.

Ancient Egyptian priests and healers believed in the sacred geometry of the universe. This consisted of "a set of mathematical ratios and proportions." They believed that these ratios, if used in the sound of music and the architecture of buildings (pyramids), would resonate with the life forces of the universe and thus enhance life.[5] Sound was a key element in ancient healing practices. Some of the pyramids, in particular one called the "house of the spirit," had sound chambers used in medical practices. The physicians would diagnose and treat the patients by using the frequency of sound waves to realign the body. These chambers were often built over waterways using various tunnels to channel the water; each patient, using their own intuition, would choose a platform

---

5 Tariq Sawandi, "Yorubic Medicine: The Art of Divine Herbology," accessed February 9, 2022, https://planetherbs.com/research-center/theory-articles/yorubic-medicine-the-art-of -divine-herbology.

AFRICAN AMERICAN HERBALISM

to stand on for this modality. The sound frequencies created by the waterways specific to the tunnel traveled upward to resonate through the crystal platforms into the body, creating realignment.[6]

Using sound as a healing agent persists in modern times. Scientific studies have shown that human thoughts could affect the structure of molecules in water,[7] and a shift in sound frequency and amplitude could affect heart cell patterns.[8] Is it no wonder that sound could affect healing? The human body is mostly made of water, and ancient Egyptians already knew and used the knowledge that sound can greatly influence our molecular structure. Maybe modern medicine is catching up to the ancient Egyptians.

SOUND HEALING IN MY OWN PRACTICE

I have always been inspired by the old ways and use the practice of infusing prayers and music—sacred sounds—into my herbal medicines. I encourage my clients to incorporate these modalities into their holistic wellness practice. The ways passed down by many of my teachers—as well as the understanding of how the power of breath, intent, and word—help connect the mind, body, and spirit—can lead us to the path of holistic health.

Sound healing has been one of the most influential modalities for my own personal healing journey. The church hymns of my youth, the sounds of nature, mantras and sound wave frequencies, as well as the beat of the drums during ceremonies—these all put me in a trance that brought me closer to myself and the most high (God), and to our ancestors. The drum is such an integral part of our ceremonies as a people.

6 See "The Pyramid Code," episode 1, which details these sound chambers.
7 See Masaru Emoto, *The Hidden Messages in Water* (New York: Atria Books, 2005).
8 See Hanae Armitage, "Sound Research: Scientific Innovations Harness Noise and Acoustics for Healing," *Stanford Medicine* (Spring 2018).

I witnessed this with my work with the late Sobonfu Somé, one of the foremost experts on African spirituality. She focused much of her work on helping heal grief within the community. She brought ceremonies from the Dagara tribe to the Western world. Her two-day ceremonies provided a way for a village to come together collectively to "hold space" for each individual's grief. I truly witnessed how important it is to move the emotional pain in the body so it does not stay "stuck" in one place; the tools in the ceremony help the waves of emotions flow through those who are grieving.

Sound finds its way into our inner being to facilitate change on a cellular level. It also activates the healing energy of the plants and the person seeking healing. Different drums and rhythms are unique to the tribe or region they come from. I can hear the difference and the unique patterns, and identify where some drumbeats originate. Haitian rhythms differ from those of different parts of Africa, and the Brazilian sounds differ too. When I was younger, I found that chanting, especially while at a crossroads (when making decisions) or low points in my life, helped me move through grief that had accumulated. Since then, I have always integrated chanting or singing into my daily practice. I use the songs of the orisha—African deities—to teach me how to honor nature and to help me in amplifying my prayers and working with the energies of nature's elemental forces. At times we may feel alone on this healing journey, but it is a lifelong process of connecting us to our ancestors and to ourselves.

Medical Papyruses

Medical papyruses are important documents that record medical information of ancient Egypt dating back to 1600 BCE. Of the possibly thousands of medical papyruses in ancient Egypt, fewer than a dozen have been discovered, and two of those are considered to be the most influential: the Ebers Papyrus and the Edwin Smith Papyrus.[9]

I find it fascinating that the ancient Egyptians and many others in the African continent already had a concept of how the body works on spiritual, energetic, and physical levels. The Ebers Papyrus describes medical issues, plant medicines, incantations for removing negative energies, ways of addressing different ailments, and even surgical procedures. The many translations and variations written by those who recorded their own practices of the papyrus have more than seven hundred formulas and folk remedies, multiple anatomical terms, and treatments for anything from mental illness to diabetes and insect bites. Appearing in these pages is information on the circulatory system, dermatology, gynecology, obstetrics, tumors, broken bones, intestinal issues, ophthalmology, and much more. The Edwin Smith Papyrus describes forty-eight surgical procedures. Examples of herbal remedies, skin treatments, and reproductive health found in these ancient texts follow.

Herbal remedies. The papyruses also described how plants were used as agents of healing (and many of the remedies have inspired herbal medicine today). Onions were used to prevent colds (a remedy passed down through the ages and still used today)—I will share an old folk medicine recipe of onion cough syrup later in this book. According to the ancients, plants and herbs with salutary effects included: garlic (*Allium sativum*) that "rids body of spirits," works as a mild laxative, helps sooth flatulence, and aids in digestion; mustard (*Sinapis alba*) that induces vomiting and relieves chest pains; opium poppies (*Papaver somniferum*) and turmeric (*Curcuma longa*) that help close open wounds; and myrrh (*Commiphora myrrha*) that relieves headaches, and soothes gums and toothaches.

9 "Ebers Papyrus," in Brittanica.com, https://www.britannica.com/topic/Ebers-papyrus; "Edwin Smith Papyrus," in Brittanica.com, https://www.britannica.com/topic/Edwin-Smith -papyrus.

Skin treatment. Because of my background in both holistic and medical aesthetics and skin care, I have also found it interesting that the ancient Egyptians had their own ways of treating skin issues. For example, the way vitiligo (a skin abnormality of uneven pigmentation) was treated involved applying a plant poultice to the skin and then exposing the skin to the sun. This would produce an inflammatory response that, when subsided, evened out the skin tone. When I think back to my clients over the span of my aesthetician career and to my personal journey with my own skin, I realize that the human race has been obsessed with "perfect" skin for such a long time. It isn't a modern issue; the techniques have just changed with the times.

Reproductive health. The ancient Egyptians were so advanced that physicians had already created an effective contraceptive, according to the Kahun Gynaecological Papyrus, which addressed women's health, gynecology, and obstetrics practices. Its contraceptive formula consisted of a mixture of acacia spikes, honey, and dates blended into paste and applied to wool. That wool was then inserted into the vagina. It has since been discovered that acacia spikes contain lactic acid, which acts as a natural spermicide.

The body-mind-spirit connection. Ancient practitioners understood that true holistic health stemmed from the synergy of all parts of ourselves. True balance cannot exist if all three parts—mind, body, and spirit—are not in harmony. Many cultures, such as Thailand with its traditional medicine and India with its Ayurvedic practices, still believe in this concept of medicine—that healing the soul (or spirit) and the mind is just as important as healing the body.

When lecturing on the subject of medical knowledge in ancient Egypt, I often reflect on how thousands of years ago, the Egyptians already knew how to read the body. Then, as I looked deeper into history, I realized that it was not just the Egyptians who contributed to ancient healing arts and herbal medicine. Many tribal nations in Africa also contributed to medical wisdom. The Nile River, which flows from south to north through eastern Africa, made connections among peoples and became a conduit for sharing, collecting, and spreading wisdom and knowledge. Going back to see our roots is like tossing a stone into a lake and seeing how the ripples radiate out.

Imhotep. Imhotep was the most well-known and the most documented medical teacher and practitioner in ancient Egypt, and he lived from 2667 to 2600 BCE. The Ebers Papyrus documents some of his diagnoses and treatment of more than two hundred diseases, and how he valued the great importance of diet, fasting, detoxing, and purging with enemas. At the time of his death, Imhotep was considered by many to have been the inventor of healing. Imhotep was eventually elevated by ancient Egyptians to being the god of medicine and healing, and the ancient Greeks and Romans identified him with the Greek god of medicine, Asclepius.

Yoruba Traditions of West Africa

The Yoruba people originate predominantly in the ancestral home of Yorubaland, now known as Nigeria, Benin, and Togo. Herbal medicine practices and song were revered in the practices of the West African Yoruba people.

Yeye Luisah Teish, a priestess in the Yoruba Lucumi tradition, an African-Cuban religion, is one of my most influential teachers on my journey to understanding who we of African descent are and how we worshiped before we came to America. Teish ("Yeye" or "mother," as she is affectionately referred to) was born in New Orleans, is an *Iyanifa* (mother of mysteries, with the knowledge to heal and perform ceremonies and divinations), and is an Oshun priestess (Oshun is a Yoruba river deity often referred to as a beautiful goddess of love, femininity, and fertility).

Teish taught me about the African versions of the Greek and Roman deities that I had loved and read so much about as a child, but calling their African counterparts "gods" is an understatement. Teish says that the orishas, as they are called, "are a personification of the natural elemental forces," and they give us information about how these forces look and move, and the colors, songs, dances, and herbs associated with them. By knowing this, she says, we can begin to understand how nature itself moves and how we work with and honor nature through ceremony.

The traditional religious practice is Ifá, which is both a religion and system of divination. In Ifá, Olodumare is the supreme being, or God, and each orisha is his manifestation in god or spirit form. There are many orishas and depending on the country you live in, the spelling of the names and the ideology of each one vary. During the transatlantic slave trade, these spiritual practices were transported to other regions in the West, creating other versions of Ifá, such as Santería in Puerto Rico and Cuba, as well as Yoruba Lucumi, which is centered in Cuba and was intertwined with Catholicism so it could be practiced. The evolution of these spiritual practices happened when we Black people had to hide our ways, adapt, and try to embrace our culture during and after the Middle Passage.

Some Yoruba traditions have over four hundred orishas, ranging from ones representing infectious diseases to the ocean goddess, who is said to help women during childbirth. There are seven major orishas (see Appendix A), but since we are talking about plants, I will add one more and focus on him: Osain, the orisha of the plants.

Teish says that according to legend, Osain and his magic are so powerful that no one can unravel his spells. Consequently, he is petitioned for any purpose where unconquerable magic is required.

Osain is often depicted as an extremely disfigured man. He has one eye, one hand, one foot, one tiny ear that can hear even a pin drop, and one ear larger than his head that hears nothing. But he can work faster, dance more beautifully, and see better than anyone because that is how many of our people view the power of the plants … powerful!

Teish taught me his song and I wept as I sang it. I HAD FINALLY FOUND MY SONG!

Never before had I felt so connected to the legacies of my plant-loving African ancestors and to how my ancestors were before—when we were on our own land and living in the old ways. The Yoruba people believe that Osain does not bless a plant you do not harvest yourself. (I feel that he is a little more open these days in our modern world of online plant medicine shopping.) Thus, at the time of the harvest, devotees of Osain—called Osainistas—would gather plants while singing the song and doing a dance. I remember the elder Teish having us all do this one-armed, one-legged dance while singing this chant:

Osain ade *(Royal Osain)*

Irerere koko *(Your blessings come first)*

I was so proud to teach this chant to everyone I met. One simple version is popular with the people of Trinidad; the words are repeated in song before harvesting the plants to ask for Osain's blessings.

Teish and other elders and teachers such as Sobonfu Some' explain that true balance and holistic health are achieved only through these practices:

* Participating in ceremonies regularly
* Using the plants as medicine and in spiritual baths
* Being in harmony with a community as well as mother earth
* Following a healthy diet
* Focusing on personal development

This is the way to achieve a balanced and joyful life.

The spiritual and medicinal use of herbs and plants is called *ewe* in the Yoruba tradition, and it is one of the most important parts of the ceremonies. There is a ceremony for almost everything. One of my greatest teachers is Sobonfu Some', a member of the Dagara tribe of Burkina Faso. Some' says that according to the ways of her tribe, you are either leaving a ceremony, preparing for the next, or thinking about future ones for certain times of the year. Ceremonies can be for anything, including rites of passage, purifying the energetic body, illnesses, connecting to the ancestors, fertility, grief, death, the greater good of the village, harvesting, and good hunting. In the lands of the Yoruba people, the herbs for these ceremonies are gathered by the priests, herbalists, and those called to them. These plants are then used in making medicines, spiritual baths for purification rituals, and decocted teas to bring about shifts in energy and health, as well as purification in bathing rituals.

In my travels and in my studies of indigenous cultures, I have found that it is only in modern conventional medicine where spiritually based herbal practices are absent or uncommon. However, they are near and dear to my practice, and I use them with each of my clients. We often forget the importance of taking care of our energetic bodies (that is, a body made up of channels of energy), and these herbal traditions help remedy that oversight.

The Impact of the Transatlantic Slave Trade on Herbalism

There is no easy way to discuss the horrors of the Middle Passage. There is also no way to speak of our history in herbalism without discussing it. We speak of it to honor the ones we lost, the ones who were enslaved, and the ones who fought for our freedom. We speak of it to shed light on and give voice to what our ancestors endured as well as to honor them for the contributions they were forced into to build the new worlds.

The Middle Passage was the forced voyage of enslaved Africans across the Atlantic Ocean to the New World. They were taken from Africa and sent to the Caribbean, and eventually to North America and South America, where they were put to work. It took anywhere from three weeks to eighty days for these captives to make this journey in packed ships. The route was named the Middle Passage because it was the middle part of a triad: One leg of the triangular trade route took goods (such as knives, guns, ammunition, cotton cloth, tools, and brass dishes) from Europe to Africa, the "middle" leg transported Africans to work as slaves in the Americas and West Indies, and the final leg took items, mostly raw materials, produced on the plantations (sugar, rice, tobacco, indigo, rum, and cotton) back to Europe.[10]

In 1807, the US Congress banned importing slaves, but the domestic trafficking and the interstate trade of enslaved people continued. Enslaved people were being moved by way of the Mississippi River to accommodate the growing cotton industry in the South; women were used for breeding to produce more bodies for work and for sale.

The bittersweet history of the American South is full of stories of the horrors endured by enslaved people, as well as of the vast amount of money made from the sale and forced labor of my people. With the slave trade, a blending of medicines and spiritual practices arose in America. This amalgam created a melting pot of immense knowledge that melded with the plant knowledge of the indigenous peoples. We created a unique way to survive and began to try to heal our people.

Often used as birthing workers and as healers for their masters' families, our people quickly became used for another aspect of their wisdom and abilities—healing. Sick enslaved people were not as valuable as healthy

10 Stephanie E. Smallwood, *Saltwater Slavery: A Middle Passage from Africa to American Diaspora* (Cambridge, MA: Harvard University Press, 2008). See "Middle Passage," in Brittanica.com, https://www.britannica.com/topic/Middle-Passage-slave-trade.

ones; therefore, healing our own was one way of protecting ourselves. You would not trust the ones who enslaved you to heal you.

We created an entire food movement called soul food—food so good it can only be described as a spiritual experience. This creation is a true embodiment of our abilities to work as alchemists, turning what seemed like nothing into something so beautiful to, again, help our own people find a form of celebration in the most difficult times of our history. We also used the plants time and time again to set us free. We used them as our weapons in war to liberate ourselves. This is also why some herbalism and certain plants became illegal, out of fear of the enslavers that the practice was and would be again used against them. I am honored to stand in the legacy of such strength and resilience and share some herbal recipes and remedies with you later in this book.

As I said before, there is no way to include all our history within these pages. I can tell only the stories the way I have heard and found them in my own journey to discovering what my people went through, who we are, and who we were as a people. This book is meant to challenge what you think you know and open up the pathways to sharing our rich and powerful history of plant medicine and the healing arts. I honor all those who came before me … let our journey through the South continue.

CHAPTER 2

THE GRANDMOTHERS OF AMERICAN HERBALISM

This chapter is of great significance to me because it honors some of the most important women in the folk tradition of the American South. There is a lack of representation of people of color in herbalism and there are very few books written by Black people and from a Black perspective about the South and its traditions. I had to search far and wide for the books I did find, and many of the ones that hold the old stories are out of print. Due to the limited written information on my people's medicines and traditions, finding the information written by a person of color is harder than you might think.

I am reminded of an old African saying: "When an elder dies, a library is burnt to the ground." Herbal folk medicine was by and large an oral tradition and not many of the remedies and practices were written down. When I interview elders about folk remedies and stories of their youth, they often talk of the old folk medicine ways and how they have died off. They simply say, "No one does it anymore like our grandmothers did; we need to come back to the old ways in order to get ourselves healthy again."

Most of the elders I meet still remember the old recipes, and when I talk about the old ways with them, they light up with excitement and start remembering things their great-grandmothers did when they were sick. It always warms my heart to share these moments so they know that our people's medicine is still out there and making a come-back. I let them know that the younger generations have not forgotten the knowledge passed down from generation to generation, that we are on a journey of coming back home. That is why I tell the stories—to honor those before us and recognize how important this folk medicine is to the history of our country.

My goal for this chapter is to also inspire you to interview your parents, grandparents, and elders, and to seek out the medicine makers' old recipes and food traditions, the healers, and the keepers of the stories in each of your communities and families. The act of preserving those stories gives you an opportunity to learn something new about your own family, ancestors, and elders. These stories are keepsakes for the future generations of your family, so they get to know where you come from and who you are on a deeper level.

You can also make people aware of the importance of ancestor rever-ence, which is the act of devotion, caring for, and honoring those who have died or, as I like to say, crossed over. We do this, first and foremost, to honor those who have come before us and ask for support, guidance, and protection. Ancestor reverence also means treasuring information we received from those who are a part of our DNA, as well from those we have chosen to be ancestors. We may ask our chosen ancestors to still be a part of us in our life journey.

Writer Alice Walker once said in an interview that the earth is full of ancestors and that most people never pay attention to this fact, making most people feel incredibly lonely. Ancestors are the ones who carry the indigenous ways; unfortunately, most do not acknowledge ancestors, discrediting what they are capable of doing. Walker also talked about how much she leans on ancestors for support and describes the feeling as an inner knowing. She said that it is almost as if we are zombies and that failure to acknowledge our ancestors makes us deeply impoverished as modern people.

I love the research I do to prepare my lectures and the stories that people gift me with. Stories are gifts because I believe they are part of who people truly are. When we stop to bear witness to people and stand in the present moment, we can connect with each other and see each other in ways that transcend our impressions of one another. To me, experiencing this is an honor—I am called, by some, a "keeper of stories" because of the incredible healing journey that these stories have led me on.

In this chapter you will read about some amazing women in history who were pivotal to the survival of their communities and carried on the traditions and remedies that had been passed down from generation to generation. These women became important to me: They shared their knowledge and confirmed how much of the story of herbalism remains untold, and—let me add a personal note here—these women become part of my herbal family.

I hope that these women will inspire you to use the plants to help bring communities together and to honor the elders by spending time with them. Our tradition also holds that speaking the names of people who are no longer on this earth makes them feel honored in the afterlife. I often say these women are my chosen ancestors, the aunties and grandmothers who have helped me become a better herbalist, healer, and community activist. Let us journey through the South and honor them. I hope this inspires you to interview some of your own people and start your own journey to be a keeper of the stories.

Herbal Remedies and Healers—
Their History in the American South

When African American people were enslaved, they depended on their traditional remedies and their own people for healing; others such as the enslavers and their harsher medicines were not to be trusted. The thinking was … you cannot be healed by the hands of the ones who hurt you.

Often, enslaved women were trained as midwives by the grandmothers of the community. These grandmothers as well as medicine women treated most people's illnesses. These female herbalists—as well as a few men—were the "keepers of the craft." Their methods spilled over into the world of the white slaveholders. Many plantation owners would use these midwives to deliver their own babies and heal from their herbal remedies.

Harsh laws regulating herbalism originated in the times of slavery of the eighteenth and nineteenth centuries. Slave revolts were occurring and sometimes the enslaved fought by using their knowledge of the plants to poison their enslavers and free themselves. Laws were enacted to restrict herbal use. Enslaved African Americans could be harshly punished, or even killed, for practicing herbal medicine or other traditions of healing. Virginia state records show that between 1780 and 1864, fifty-eight enslaved people were convicted of poisoning or attempted poisoning.[11] In October 1748, Virginia passed a law that forbade Black people from preparing or administering medicine. Doing so would be a felony and could be punishable by death. By 1792 the law was amended because whites wanted to use Black people for healing as long as these healers were monitored and had good intentions. In 1843 it was amended again to allow Black healers to sell medicine under the

---

11 Wyndham Bolling Blanton, *Medicine in Virginia in the 18th Century* (University of Michigan: Garrett & Massie, 1931), 174.

AFRICAN AMERICAN HERBALISM

watchful eye of their masters. Between 1748 and 1884, many Black healers and herbalists were brought to trial for practicing medicine illegally, but only the enslaved person would be punished while their masters could use them for services as they pleased. These practices were designed to control the way the Black healers would practice.[12]

The Civil War ended slavery in 1865, but even though the Fourteenth Amendment conferred Black citizens equal protection under the law, difficult times were ahead. What took root was Jim Crow, the racial caste system that operated primarily in the American South and border states, between 1877 and the mid-1960s. The US Supreme Court case *Plessy v. Ferguson* (1896) gave the legal imprimatur to Jim Crow laws and the Jim Crow way of life—racial segregation and dehumanization of Black people. Voting restrictions became an issue all over the South. In 1896, Louisiana had 130,334 registered Black voters. In just eight years, that number would dwindle down to only 1,342. Only 1 percent could pass the state's new rules. Separate schools, separate public accommodations, separate drinking fountains and toilets—it was a system designed to stamp the badge of inferiority on Black citizens kept in place by white violence.[13, 14, 15]

12 Todd L. Savitt, "Influence of Slave Healers," in *Medicine and Slavery: The Diseases and Health Care of Blacks in Antebellum Virginia* (Urbana, IL: University of Illinois Press, 1978), 143.
13 Jim Crow laws affected every aspect of Black people's lives all over the country. In Los Angeles, Black people could not enter white stores. After World War I, Black soldiers came home to lynching even while they were wearing their uniforms. "A Brief History of Jim Crow," Constitutional Rights Foundation, https://www.crf-usa.org/black-history-month/a-brief-history-of-jim-crow.
14 Black men could not shake hands with white men because that would suggest that they were equals. They could also not comment, approach, or provide any services to white women lest they risk being accused of rape. Black people could not ride in cars with whites unless they sat in the back, and on the road whites would have right of way. Certain "etiquette" rules were also added: whites would have to be addressed as "Mr." or "Mrs." while Blacks could be addressed only by their first name. David, Pilgrim, "What Was Jim Crow," Ferris State University, https://www.ferris.edu/HTMLS/news/jimcrow/what.htm.
15 Lynchings, rapes, and arson would also become common as whites kept retaliating. It happened on a large scale in the Tulsa Massacre on May 31 and June 1, 1921, which began because a young Black male rode an elevator with a white woman and was accused of rape.

After slavery ended, however, many women set up their herbal businesses closest to the plants they already knew about and in the towns nearest to them. They would continue to honor the midwife and medicine-making traditions to keep their families alive and thriving while helping their communities as well.

Through the stories of these grandmothers and others, I have learned herbalism was alive and thriving, especially in rural areas of the South. Due to lack of money, hospitals (especially for people of color), and transportation, people in rural areas found it difficult to get medical care from doctors or hospitals.[16]

Also, most people were in the practice of not trusting anyone outside their communities, especially with things that seemed new to them, such as modern medicine. They had always relied on folk medicine as their primary healing modality. As farmers and people of the earth, they would trust only things from the earth at that time.

But it was not only people in the community who relied on these healers. Around the 1930s medical doctors pushed back against the herbalists because the doctors were finding it difficult to attract patients. Why? Because most people in the community already trusted these "granny midwives" or "granny women"—those Black female midwives, healers, and herbalists in the American South—making it almost impossible for the medical doctors to practice because of the lack of patients.

What I have learned from these stories is how important these women are to the history of herbalism. Most risked jail and even death to practice their craft tirelessly and sometimes without payment, just to be of service. I want to show how African Americans have used plants to

Around three hundred people were killed. Tulsa Historical Society & Museum, https://www.tulsahistory.org.

16 Swannanoa Valley Museum, "Catching Babies: Midwife Mary Stepp Burnette Hayden," Swannanoa Valley Museum & History Center, April 23, 2018, https://www.history.swannanoavalleymuseum.org/catching-babies-midwife-mary-stepp-burnette-hayden.

turn toward—instead of away from—each other. These women treated everyone, no matter if they had money or were of another race. There are so many amazing medicine people, but as I have said, I can speak about only a few in these pages. Each of these women has inspired me as a practitioner, herbalist, and person in my community. I hope their stories will inspire your journey with the plants and encourage you to share your knowledge with your communities.

Emma Dupree "Lil Medicine Thang"

"All that we see, everything that is growin' in the earth, is healin' to the nation of any kind of disease."

~Emma Dupree

Emma Dupree (July 4, 1897–March 12, 1996) was one of seven children of Pennia and Noah Williams, formerly enslaved but free at the time of Dupree's birth. Dupree grew up on a farm near Falkland, North Carolina. She eventually had two husbands and five children. Her first marriage, at age twenty, to Ethan Cherry, lasted a year: As the story goes, "that Cherry went one wisecrack too far about how many women it takes to satisfy a man. Dupree whacked him with a chair. Knocked him out cold. Then she divorced him. 'He wasn't no good husband.'" Dupree then married Austin Dupree.[17]

Dupree got her nickname "'Lil Medicine Thang" because of her love of nature and foraging in the woods. She had been an herbalist and medi-

---

17 Paige Williams, "Herbalist, 94, Lets Nature Heal," *Tulsa World*, last updated February 25, 2019, https://tulsaworld.com/archive/herbalist-94-lets-nature-heal/article_3b0e06d1-4af9-5567-93ee-bc4b50d5867f.html.

cine woman since she was a child, when she began collecting plants near the Tar River area. While other children played, she would be picking herbs and roots. She truly reminds me of myself as a child—collecting plants, mixing things, eating them, and making my brother also try my "medicines." I laugh when I say that my brother was my first herbal client. The elders in Dupree's community would comment about her love for the plants, saying that she was always harvesting something. Eventually, they began to call her by that nickname, asking what is that "little medicine thang doing now?"

Dupree said in many interviews that God taught her the plants and that is how she had such a deep connection so early in life to the plant world. Her saying this reminds me of an expression, "THEY ARE A PLANT," which is what I say when I know that I have found a plant teacher. This means that the plant world has accepted the plant teacher and whatever plant they would choose would produce healing medicine. Plant teachers are truly connected to the earth and have an inner knowledge of the earth's secrets. Dupree was just that person. But she also explored the world outside herbal medicine. Later in life, she interned with a medical doctor to further her knowledge of the medical and plant worlds so she could be a better practitioner.

When I researched the plants she used, I was always intrigued by her herbal formulations and the way she would use them. Some would say that the concoctions looked like tobacco juice and smelled like turpentine. Dupree had a famous nine-herb tonic that is still talked about today. Unfortunately, this recipe is lost to us, but I am on a quest to find it!

I was fascinated when I saw how her use of plants differed from how "modern" herb books and teachers would talk about using certain plants. I learned that she just had her own special connection to the plants and a unique way of healing people. I also found through many elders that people used what they had access to and therefore developed different relationships with those plants. Now plant medicine is so much more accessible.

I often close my eyes and imagine what a visit with her would have been like. Going down a dirt road, walking through her garden apothecary, and then coming up to the porch of her tiny house, all the while smelling her herbal brews that would be cooking over an open fire—that's what I dream of.

I imagine her offering me water or whatever tea she brewed for the day (Southern hospitality is a big thing). I see myself taking a seat on the porch and, after all the Southern formalities of asking about how my family is doing, she would begin to ask about what ailed me (Southern for what is going on health wise). Another part of the personality of "Aunt Emma" (as she was affectionately called by many) was her gift of presence that made your time with her a time of healing. She had the gift of making your day or problem feel better. When I heard about these qualities, I knew that she was more than an herbalist but was also a true healer—someone who helps heal the body, mind, and spirit.

As Aunt Emma would tell it, she was just the person who makes the medicine. She would say, "It is God that does the healin'." Her prescriptions would always end with a note to take the medicine with faith and prayer.

In a videotaped interview, Dupree gives a tour of her herbal apothecary garden, and she explains how she uses the plants and tells stories about her clients. This tour gives us a window to her plant world and her herbal remedies at a time when many herbalists' remedies were not documented. We learn that she used local natural resources that included plants and trees she received as gifts. Dupree tells of myriad plants: bark of sweet gum; white mint (she loved mint as a medicine and grew three different kinds); mullen (often using the tea for swollen feet and knees to "draw out the fluid"); sassafras; poke root and leaf (often called poke "salat" in the South); "rabbit tobacco" (a.k.a. life everlasting, a very important plant to our people); sage (in tea to help with stomach ulcers); and silkweed (for high blood pressure). Then there was horseradish, which she used to quell fevers by placing the leaves on the head, to calm coughs by putting the leaves on the chest, or to lower high blood pressure by making the leaves into a compress with a little Epsom salt and vinegar and putting it on the head. Dupree also had stories about clients who said her medicines helped them.

Other folk remedies we hear about in the video include smoking jimson weed for asthma and applying oil from turtle fat as a topical salve for rheumatoid arthritis. Dupree also talked about her "healing berry tree." She said she read about it in the Bible and did not know it by any other name. She said she once gave this medicine to a woman who had been told by doctors that she "had sugar" or what the old folks in the South call diabetes. Dupree "packed up a jar," meaning she placed the berries in a mason jar along with brown sugar, rock candy, honey, or whatever sweetener she had on her at the time, and that mixture would draw out the power of the plant.

Dupree also talked about using wild cherries (with the leaves) soaked in a sweetener like molasses or honey as blood tonics to purify or nourish the blood. Keeping the blood healthy is an important part of African American herbal medicine practices to this day. She truly believed in the power of the plants and would proudly state her age with a little swirl in her step and then talk about how healthy and full of energy she was because of them.

Dupree's additional remedies include a white mint potion for poor circulation; catnip tea for babies with colic; tansy tea—hot or cold—for low blood sugar; and mullein tea for a stomachache. She often would mix her remedies with molasses, sugar, peppermint, or rock candy to knock out the bitterness of the herbs when needed.

Dupree also spoke of her concern about the purity of our water systems. Noting the dirty, rusty pipes in homes, she encouraged people to think about all of the things that go in their body because what we put in us circulates all through us. Food and proper cooking practices were important to her. She believed food and herbs that accent it should be our medicine, that those are the agents of healing and preventing illnesses. Dupree would comment that people "didn't cook things right anymore" and that adding plant medicine made food healthier and easier to digest.[18]

With her deep faith in God, Dupree would credit all her work as coming through God because God created all that we have on earth. She would say she could talk to you for hours but eventually, she would say, it would be His words that she would speak.

Thank you, Aunt Emma, for your work, your inspiration to help us connect more deeply to each other and to all things around us and above us, and for the knowledge that the love of the plant world is a true calling.

Mary Stepp Burnette Hayden

When I first discovered Mary Hayden in my quest to learn more about the stories of African American herbalism, her granddaughter Mary Othella Burnette was one of the first people to step forward. I was living in Asheville, North Carolina, when I learned that one of the most important people in herbalism and midwifery history had lived right there. Then something happened—I'm not sure what—and I began to randomly get connected with some of Hayden's

18 "Little Medicine Thing: Emma Dupree, Herbalist," interview by the Office of Health Services Research and Development, School of Medicine, East Carolina University, 1979, audio, 34:55, https://digital.lib.ecu.edu/58575.

relatives, including Mary Othella Burnette. I was thrilled to interview Burnette, and our subsequent correspondence was what got me through the beginning of the COVID-19 pandemic.

I hold in very high regard the privilege of being able to interview the elders. Burnette and I exchanged a few emails until we could pick a day to talk to each other on the phone. And oh did we talk. She graced me with so many stories about what it was like for African Americans growing up in the South. I could hear in her voice the excitement and pride as she talked about the Black history of southern Appalachia. I just let her talk and say what she needed to stay (if you ever interview the elders, it is so important to just let them speak).

Burnette gifted me with her warm presence, knowledge, and excitement of being able to share these stories of the South and of her herbalist grandmother Mary Hayden and all the work that she did in western North Carolina. This is her story.

Mary Hayden, as Burnette tells it, was born during the time of slavery, in January 1858, to Hanah Stepp on the Joe Stepp farm in Black Mountain, North Carolina. Family lore has it that when Hayden was around five years old, a man on a horse came up to her house and read the Emancipation Proclamation and told them that they were free.

Hayden grew up to be small, maybe a hundred pounds, but sturdy. She was part Native American and spoke a different dialect. She had long hair and would wear it in two braids wrapped around her head. She always wore a handmade apron and would put all her things in it, including herbs and materials she foraged to make medicine for the community.

Said Burnette: Granny told me that "every herb has three kinds—one is a healer, one is just a weed, and the other is a poison. Meaning one is positive, one is neutral, and one is negative."

Hayden was more than just an herbalist. Her mother, a midwife, taught her to deliver and care for babies. Eventually, Hayden became the midwife for most of the county—probably the first African American women registered as a midwife in the county, says Burnette—and she continued working until she was well into her eighties.

Hayden was a familiar figure in the area. She would leave at night, said Burnette, no matter what time it was, carrying her lantern with her supplies, and journey over the mountain to birth babies of any race. Sometimes she would be awake all night long during a birth. Some of these expeditions were harrowing, like when Hayden was chased by a large wild cat because it had gotten a whiff of the large ham Hayden had just received as payment for delivering a baby.

Hayden was such an important part of western North Carolina's history. She was one of those women who held together communities. For example, when midwifery began to be restricted by law in the 1920s, these restrictions adversely affected people of color, most of whom were poor and lacked access to doctors and hospitals. Hayden made sure to get sterile birthing supplies from the county so she could continue to provide services to her community safely, Burnette said.

I was touched when Burnette told me that she, too, was birthed by her own grandmother Mary Hayden. It was beautiful to know that she was a part of a legacy.

I am blessed to have gotten to know more about Burnette. She told stories that I had never heard before about the traditions and day-to-day life of the South and how the races comingled. We also talked shop: Burnette remembered the herbal remedies used in her family and those that her grandmother used for the community. The ones Burnette was most excited about were the tansy tea and ground ivy. When she would speak about ground ivy and drinking the tea, you could hear the nostalgia in her voice. I told her about how I had to learn to love ground ivy from all my years of gardening and my internships. And—hey—we also swapped recipes.

Burnette helped me realize that the stories of African Americans have been omitted, that there are many perspectives, and that it is so important for us to preserve these stories for future generations. Since our time together, she has written about her life in the South in *Lige of the Black Walnut Tree: Growing Up Black in Southern Appalachia*.

Thank you, Mary Hayden, for all your work in continuing the legacy of our grandmothers' grandmothers, for healing her community, and fighting to keep midwives in practice. You were always of service to everyone. Also I honor her granddaughter Mary Othella Burnette for helping protect and share these stories for future generations.

Henrietta Jeffries

The story of Henrietta Jeffries inspired me to appreciate what happens when the community stands up for itself to support one another and recognize the challenges midwives faced from the often hostile medical establishment and government. Jeffries was born to enslaved parents Elijah Phelps and Charlotte Ann Bennett, a midwife, on January 5, 1857, in Halifax County, Virginia. She eventually married and had eighteen children.[19] She made her name as a midwife more than as an herbalist. The 1910 census lists her occupation as "doctoress," or midwife, delivering both African American and white babies.

In 1911, Jeffries was put on trial for practicing medicine without a license and, if convicted, faced death by hanging. The trial made a big splash both locally and nationally when a jury of twelve white males found her guilty. Then the community gathered in the courtroom. After

19 "Caswell County Family Tree," RootsWeb, updated October 14, 2019, https://wc.rootsweb.com/trees/117534/I56628/-/individual.

AFRICAN AMERICAN HERBALISM

the verdict was read, Judge Charles M. Cooke asked who in that court-room had been birthed by her, and almost everyone stood up (some believe the judge too had been delivered by Jeffries). Here are excerpts from that conversation between Jeffries and the judge.

Sitting near the judge in the witness chair, Henrietta Jeffries waited. The judge continued: "Aunt Henrietta, it looks like it's going to be bad weather. I speck it will snow or sleet tonight, if the night is bad and it snows, the snow will fall around your humble cabin. Or maybe the sleet will beat on the roof. And just when you get warm in bed you'll hear a knocking at the door, and you'll say "Who dar?" And the voice will come to you through the storm, "Mrs. Smith is might sick and she wants you to come to her at once." What would you do, Aunt Henrietta?"

"Judge, I would get up and go." "Yes," said the judge, "I know you would. I can see you now as you pulled to your bedside with your cane, your old, ragged socks, and fastening your shawl about you, then get up behind the messenger and ride away into the night on your mission, and may God bless you, and He will. Now there is one thing I would warn you from doing. You must not give any of those women to whom you are called any medi-cine. You don't know anything about the actions of drugs. Now I don't mean that you shouldn't give them some turpentine and ditney tea, for these are about the best medicines in the world. I want to shake your hand, Aunt Henrietta So good-bye, and God spare you long to bless humankind." Then Judge Cooke turned to the clerk and said: "Mr. Clerk, take this judgment: 'In the case of State vs. Henrietta Jeffries,' the defendant is not guilty."[20]

---

20 William S. Powell, *When the Past Refused to Die: A History of Caswell County, North Carolina, 1777–1977* (Durham, NC: Moore Publishing Co., 1977), 534–537. See "Midwife on Trial\ the Descendants of a Turn-of-the-Century Midwife Will Gather to Reenact Her 1911 Trial on Charges of Practicing Medicine Without a License," updated January 28, 2015, *Greensboro News and Record,* https://greensboro.com/midwife-on-trial-the-descendants-of-a-turn-of-the -century-midwife-will-gather-to/article_25982df4-4a94-5baf-8709-63ff159bec28.html.

The judge dismissed all charges. Black people in those times rarely had the influence of Jeffries, who had delivered most of the babies in that community. Her acquittal meant that she was free to deliver babies, which she did well into her later years. Her family has preserved her legacy by providing information on her life and times.

Thank you, Henrietta Jeffries, for your strength and dedication to the tradition and your community, and thank you for risking your life to provide health care to the ones who needed it.

Mary Cooley

Mary Cooley was born Mary Frances Hill on August 15, 1900, in Baker County, Georgia. She eventually married a carpenter, Ashley Cooley, and moved to Albany, Georgia, in 1930. She was trained as a midwife by apprenticing with the renowned Alabama midwife Onnie Lee Logan. Cooley delivered more than three thousand babies and was known for working with both Black and white families in the segregated South. What I love most about Miss Mary Cooley is that she created an environment where the entire family could witness the birthing.

Cooley is the subject of a 1952 documentary, "All My Babies," by George Stoney. Cooley was shown making the rounds and preparing and delivering babies at people's homes. The film shows what life was like in the Georgia of the 1950s, when medical doctors were often at odds with midwifery. Despite this push by the doctors against midwives, the Georgia Health Department used the film as a training video.

One of the amusing parts of the video is seeing Cooley taking part in a training session during which a young nurse tries to teach her how to wrap an umbilical cord. Cooley's facial expression is priceless: She all but rolls her eyes, as if she's thinking, Who are they to teach someone who has delivered three thousand babies anything about catching babies?

("Catching babies" means birthing children; it is an old Southern term that midwives use.)

The video gives us an inside view of what it was like to be a midwife back in the day and what it was like when the modern medical world crossed paths with traditional midwifery. Cooley would participate in prenatal care as well as postpartum care. She would bring food or do anything that each family needed, including cleaning and cooking, so that the mothers could rest. Cooley would tirelessly work after hours and around the clock to make sure that her clients were well taken care of body, mind, and soul.

I honor Mary Cooley for the work she did in inspiring others to take a better approach to prenatal and postnatal care. She provided all-around care for her patients, using the ways of our people and inspiring others to do the same. Her work helped bridge the gap between the worlds of modern medicine and folk medicine.

Onnie Lee Logan

Born around 1910 in Sweet Water, Alabama, Onnie Lee Logan was the daughter of landowners at a time when it was way more common for African Americans to be sharecroppers. Logan was very feisty and was devoted to what she said she was called to do as a teacher of midwifery and herbal medicine to many in her community. Logan was a bridge between the spiritual and medical practice of midwifery. She also used old folk traditions, such as putting a knife under the bed during labor to symbolically cut the pain of childbirth—which is something my grandmother talked about too.

Logan tells about her experiences in *Motherwit: An Alabama Midwife's Story,* in which she noted that she was forgetting many things and wanted to preserve them in a book. The title "motherwit" describes herself and her education classes for new and expecting parents. "There was a higher power and God give me wisdom. Motherwit, common sense. Wisdom come from on high. You got it and you cain't explain how you got it yo' self. It's motherwit."[21] The book explains some of her practices, such as using hot towels to help with dilation during birthing.

Herbs and folk healing traditions she used included mullein leaves, used as poultices to lessen swelling of the feet during pregnancy. Another tradition was preparing a tea made from steeping a man's sweaty shirt so it could be sipped to "sweat out" a fever (Boneset herb tea was good for that too). She also believed that if a child suffered from asthma, the remedy involved taking the child to the woods and pounding a nail into a pine tree above the child's head; as the child grew, the ailment would transfer itself into the tree.

As I was growing up in the South, so many practices—called "old wives' tales"—were what children and adults just did because the elders told us to. I honestly believe in many of them to this day. In my opinion, maybe it was the ceremony and power of intent more than the exact action itself that brought about the healing.

It was not until 1976 that Alabama outlawed lay midwives. Onnie Lee Logan, however, was one of the last midwives in Mobile, Alabama, and she was allowed to continue to practice until 1984. She passed away in 1995.

Ms. Onnie, thank you for your feisty spirit that helped you continue to practice the craft, and for leaving your words to inspire many on the path to midwifery. Thank you for creating ceremonies that brought faith and spirit to the practice of health and wellness.

---

21 Onnie Lee Logan, *Motherwit: An Alabama Midwife's Story* (San Francisco, CA: Untreed Reads, 2013).

CHAPTER 3

THE PLANT WORLD

I have spent my entire life with plants. I grew up on a farm, and I spent all my time outside. My first plant ally was the passionflower, or maypop, as it is called in the South, but I did not realize it was an ally at first. Here's what happened. One day during one of my herbal medicine internships, we were in the garden harvesting passionflowers when one of the pods popped open and I smelled the aroma of my childhood. So many emotions came over me as I realized how long the plants had been with me for my own healing. I lay in the vines and stared at the alienlike flowers and popped the pods just to smell them. I realized that day that the plants have always spoken to me, telling me of their medicine and asking me to see them.

I grew up on folk medicine: whenever anything bad happened, the plants and those old-timey remedies were there for me. I feel blessed to have grown up in the craft and often laugh about how this has truly become my life, when in my teenage years I had just wanted to be a city girl and get out of the garden! Now I feel most at peace if I am surrounded by the plant world and nature. Believe me. If I am outside, I am looking at the ground and around me, trying to find medicine and telling people, "Oh, that is good for … "

My journeys called me back home to the mountains, red dirt, rivers, and pine trees of my youth. I wanted to stay put and learn the medicines and stories of the South, my native land. I realized it was my purpose in life to work with plants and share this knowledge.

There are many ways to study herbalism, even if you just want to learn to help yourself and your family first. Then, after more training, you can reach out to your community, but I believe it is important to start with the plants nearby. Here's what two North Carolina herbalists say about using plants in their lives, a skill that they learned from the elders and their stories, and from oral tradition.[22]

Sally McCloud on Foraging, Making Medicine

We used boneset for colds ... It's kinda a real thin weed ... calamus for colds too ... I just mix it all together and it's good for colds ... Boneset, calamus, and yellow root ... If I get one first, then I save it until I can find the other ones ... When I get all three of 'em ... I put them together then boil it and strain it out, sit it in the Frigidaire and I drink it when I need it. ... Catnip was fer if you had a fever, boil it and then drink it.[23]

Ruth Patterson on Catnip, Goldenrod

I always raise catnip around my house. If the baby had colic, get dat catnip and boil it. Take a teaspoon full of dat catnip and put it in a li'l cup and squeeze some milk out yo breast in dat cup wit dat catnip tea. Den take a li'l bitty spoon and let it drip off of dat spoon in dat baby mouth and won't have no colic. Them goldenrod is good for colds. It's got a leaf bought yeah long, look like a sage leaf, only it's shiny and it has a heap

22 Michele Elizabeth Lee, *Working the Roots: Over 400 Years of Traditional African American Healing* (Laurel Hill, NC: Wadastick Publishers, 2017).
23 Lee, *Working the Roots*, 9.

of leaves grows up on it, and the stem goes straight up, jus bout dat high. I ain't never had a cold. I drank dat yellow root water twice a day.[24]

Foraging and Wildcrafting

I want to invite you into your own surroundings. I feel it is the best way to start learning about the plants in your own backyard. Mother Nature gives us what we need if we can just open ourselves up and look. Each season I look around me to see what plants are most prolific, and the plants tell me what I will be battling for the next season.

Right before the COVID-19 pandemic, I saw on my porch a baby mullein plant starting to grow out of nowhere. I had never planted it or had the seeds. It was in a pot that last season's plant had died in. Mullein is used for the respiratory system. I have always used and suggested it for use in teas and smoking blends for respiratory issues. I sat there staring at her and asking, What are you doing here?

Lately, foraging has become popular. It takes time to learn, so be patient. For me, it has been a lifelong practice. You do not have to live near nature to take part; in the city it is called urban foraging. Foraging, both urban and rural, is the practice of collecting and identifying wild foods such as tree nuts, plant roots, mushrooms, herbs, and even flowers that grow around your yard, in the forest, or on a city block. You can find plant medicine everywhere. While living in New Orleans, I found elderberries everywhere in the city.

Proceed with caution. I suggest seeking out people in your area or attending a few conferences that sponsor plant walks to help you identify what you are collecting. Do not just rely on TikTok and YouTube videos. I have seen people on social media mistake pokeberries for elderberries and making "elderberry" syrup with them. That mistake could truly poison someone.

---

24 Lee, *Working the Roots*, 93–94.

It is so exciting when you can identify a few plants. Before you know it, you will impress yourself with your knowledge.

Herb Schools and Classes

I believe what most of the elders, my herbal teachers, and colleagues know—that to be a good herbalist, you do not need to know all the plants. If you learn about ten plants well and how to use them in multiple ways, then you have a great foundation as an herbalist.

There are even schools online, but I truly believe that you need to be with the plants to learn about them. You do not have to want to be a professional herbalist to participate in these programs. All you have to be is an herb enthusiast. You can take classes on specific herbal topics; or you can do internships or apprenticeships, which has been most useful for me.

Plant Spirit Meditation

One of my favorite ways to learn about plants is through plant spirit meditation. It is the practice of taking "journeys" with the plants by taking the plant medicine or sitting with the plant in a meditative state and having the plant tell you about its medicine and magic. I used to practice this in a group years ago when I was taking an herbal internship. We never knew what we were taking. We just had to have our experience and try to guess what the plant was at the end, and everyone shared their experience.

I once took an elderberry for plant meditation; this plant is used for its antiviral properties. I had a vision of a double helix and something was trying to penetrate it. Then I saw the plant blocking it; I knew what an elderberry did at the time but not exactly how that plant did it. After that experience, my teacher said that my time with the group was finished, that I knew what I needed to know, and that the plants would teach me the rest.

There are no resources that I know of on this subject. Each person can have a unique healing and educational journey on their own. I have seen people come to a deep awareness of where their grief lies just by taking a journey with a mimosa tree tincture. Sometimes there is no need to approach psychedelic ones (which have become extremely popular lately) when all plants can lead you back to yourself. I use this technique in combination with other modalities in my grief and other healing ceremonies to help people release and go deeper into those areas that need extra love and attention.

How to Journey with the Plants

Find the plant that you want to study either in tea or tincture form (I prefer tincture), or find it growing and take a little while sitting with it. Both combined are powerful!

Take a dropperful of the tincture and get into a comfortable position; have a pen and paper handy to take notes about your experience.

Allow twenty or so minutes by setting your timer.

Do you notice any changes and sensations in your body? Does it get warm or cool? Do you feel the medicine in certain parts? Do you notice colors or see images? Do not judge your journey or wonder if you are doing it correctly; just try to disconnect, breathe deeply, and experience. Take time to write about it.

Then look up the plant in a book and compare your notes.

Remember—all of us have ancestors who used plant medicine to survive. None of us would be here if that were not true. Sometimes it just takes us to reconnect, to call back in the knowledge of our ancestors. The knowledge of plants is truly in your bone marrow as I have learned from my own experiences with farming and remembering what was used when I was young.

Growing Your Own Plants

One of the best ways to learn is to just grow a plant. There is something about watching a plant grow from a seed, harvesting it, and then making it into a plant medicine. This cycle of life is truly an all-inclusive learning experience.

After disconnecting from the practices of my youth and getting lost in my life, I was even afraid of killing a fake plant. One day, an elder said, "Just put some seeds in the earth and see what happens." I replied, "I come from farmers and plant people." So that is exactly what I did, and I called on my ancestors to help guide me. At first, I was the overdressed girl with the cute purse. Then one pot became two, one patch became a garden. Because I learned so much from the old farmers and herb growers, now I am the girl who keeps dirty rain boots in her car so if I

AFRICAN AMERICAN HERBALISM

see something or hear the plants calling, I can just stop the car and go to them in the woods.

If you are just starting out, you do not even need land—you can just buy baby plants. To learn more about farming and gardening, check out *Farming While Black*[25] or attend local gardening or farming classes.

The Plants

Here are descriptions of some of the plants used in the South, as well as some of my favorite medicinal plants, along with botanical drawings to help you understand them.[26] I detail only a few of the many, many plants used by herbalists. According to the Audubon Society of North Carolina, in the state where I am from, there are over four thousand native plant species. We are so lucky that Mother Nature loves us so much, but as you can see, it is a lifelong process to learn about even a portion of the plant world. For some of you, this will be the beginning of a journey to learn the plants.

Note: This information on plant medicine in this book is for reference only. It should not be used to diagnose and treat illnesses or prescribe treatment. Consult a medical practitioner for health advice before trying any new herbal protocols.

Note: A typical rule of thumb for the "magical rootwork element" of each plant is that what they do medicinally they can also do magically. Rootworkers are a type of traditional healer and conjurer (workers of magic) of the rural, Black South. They use herbal plants, roots, potions,

25 Leah Penniman, *Farming While Black: Soul Fire Farm's Practical Guide to Liberation on the Land,* (Hartford, VT: Chelsea Green Publishing, 2018).

26 Thomas Easley and Steven Horne, *The Modern Herbal Dispensatory: A Medicine Making Guide* (Berkeley, CA: North Atlantic Books, 2016); Darryl Patton, *Mountain Medicine: The Herbal Remedies of Tommie Bass* (Miami, FL: Little River Press, 2017); Michele L. Lee, *Working the Roots: Over 400 Years of African American Healing* (Sacramento, CA: Wadastick Publishing, 2017).

and spells in various forms to assist a person in what they require for healing or other matters.

Aloe (*Aloe vera*)

Traditional Uses: Soothes irritated or dry skin, mucous membranes, burns, and other damaged tissues; heals cuts; soothes cracked, dry nipples during nursing; has a cooling effect; clears constipation and moves the bowels; cools and invigorates the blood; promotes menses; helps digestion; and kills internal parasites.

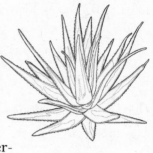
Aloe

Contraindications: Some herbalists suggest that children, the elderly, or pregnant or nursing women should not consume aloe vera juice internally. However, this warning may apply only to the green outer leaf or to aloe vera concentrates. Consuming small amounts of diluted pulp juice is typically found not to be harmful. Do not apply topically to wounds with staph infections.

Magical Rootwork Elements: Stops gossip about you, protects against enemies or negative influences.

Bay Leaf (*Laurus nobilis*)

Traditional Uses: Used as a nervine to calm the nervous system; used to treat fevers and arthritis; repels insects; used by both Native and African Americans to treat colds, flu, and congestion; often used as a poultice placed on an affected area for treatment or in a bath to relieve pain and inflammation.

Contraindications: May interfere with blood sugar.

Magical Rootwork Elements: Protects against bad energy or ill intent; burning leaves with words written on them that describe your heart's desire has been a longtime practice; as an incense, helps with protection and clearing the negative energy—the elders taught me this. I use bay leaves also in many spiritual bath formulas when I am trying to call things I desire or need into my life.

Black Cohosh *(Cimicifuga racemose or Actae racmosa)*

Traditional Uses: Alleviates hot flashes, menopause symptoms, irregular menstruation, PMS (premenstrual syndrome); used as a nervine (to calm the nervous system); used to treat bronchitis and coughs; is an anti-inflammatory; is anti-spasmodic; is mildly analgesic; lowers blood pressure; purifies blood; used by Native people for treating venomous bites and stings.

Contraindications: Stimulates uterine contractions, so its use is not advised in early pregnancy. Be careful if you are breastfeeding, heavily menstruating, or have a family history of so-called female cancers (gynecologic cancers such as cervical, ovarian, uterine, vaginal, vulvar, and the very rare fallopian tube cancer); in large doses, black cohosh can cause headaches, dizziness, irritation of the central nervous system, nausea, and vomiting. It is best used as a small part of a formula and with the guidance of a health professional.

Magical Rootwork Elements: For courage and protection; also assists in drawing love to you, to help pull negative energy up and out of the body.

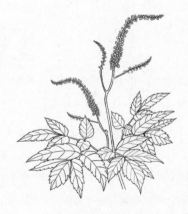

Black Cohosh

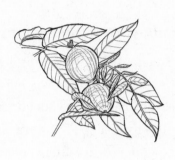
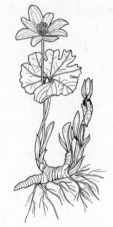

Black Walnut   Bloodroot or "Coon Root"

Black Walnut (*Juglans nigra*)

Traditional Uses: Helps soothe and treat athlete's foot, ringworm, boils, infected wounds, mouth ulcers, canker sores, fungal infections, internal parasites, thrush, gastric candida overgrowth, and hypothyroidism; builds tooth enamel when used as a tooth powder.

Contraindications: Some people may show skin sensitivity; green hulls temporarily stain the skin; not recommended for use during pregnancy.

Magical Rootwork Elements: Used in spiritual bathing to cut ties with relationships that are no longer desired.

Bloodroot or "Coon Root" (*Sanguinaria canadensis*)

Traditional Uses: Used topically in a paste to help heal skin disorders, warts, venereal sores; used to promote coughing as stimulating expectorant for asthma, bronchitis, coughs, chronic lung infections; very powerful lymph-moving herb.

Contraindications: Small amounts may cause tunnel vision; large doses can cause nausea, vomiting, headaches, and respiratory failure. Do not use during pregnancy. People have died after using the resin incorrectly. It is recommended for use only under professional/highly knowledgeable supervision.

Magical Rootwork Elements: Offers hex breaking and protection from negative energy.

Calamus Root (*Acorus calamus*)

Traditional Uses: Helps with lung and digestive issues, colds, flu, bronchitis, and coughs by eliminating phlegm; works as a digestive aid by relieving gas, bloating, gastritis, heartburn, nausea, headaches, arthritis, sore throats, asthma, and allergies; stimulates appetite and energy; regulates menstruation; is an aphrodisiac and relaxant.

Contraindications: Pregnant and nursing women should not use a calamus root herbal supplement, as it is considered to be a uterine stimulant. Overuse (many times the recommended dosage) should be avoided, as it may cause vomiting and further serious problems; may be harmful if consumed for an extended time period.

Magical Rootwork Elements: Used to control a person or situation, often in love spells as well as other matters for them to work better in your favor; used for "uncrossing hexes."

Castor Plant (*Ricinus communis*)

Traditional Uses: Strengthens the immune system, prevents illness; is anti-inflammatory; alleviates arthritis and rheumatism when used topically; alleviates yeast infections, constipation, gastrointestinal prob-

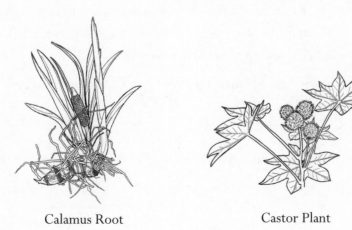

Calamus Root   Castor Plant

lems, menstrual disorders, migraines, acne, sunburn, athlete's foot, and ringworm; detoxifies; eliminates lymphatic congestion when used topically with packs or poultices (placing cotton cloth soaked in oil on the afflicted area and covering it with a towel and then adding heat); increases white blood cells; soothes skin abrasions; induces labor.

Contraindications: Do not use while pregnant, and do not take internally for more than three days. Seek medical advice before using any new herbs.

Magical Rootwork Elements: Helps things move quicker.

Catnip (*Nepeta cataria*)

Traditional Uses: Calms nerves, helps with sleep and is antispasmodic; settles the stomach and cramps; is diaphoretic (opens the pores and may promote moistening skin; helps release heat from fevers or promotes sweating); alleviates hives; helps soothe colic and teething issues; helps fight fever, measles, chicken pox, colds, chills, congestion, sore throat, and indigestion. Drinking it in tea is the best way to use this herb.

Catnip

Contraindications: Small children should not use it for extended periods of time. It can have a narcoticlike effect if overused. As with all members of the mint family, avoid use while pregnant, especially in the first trimester, as catnip may cause miscarriage.

Magical Rootwork Elements: Promotes happiness; makes women enticing to men; draws in love.

Cedar (*Juniperus virginiana*)

Traditional Uses: Helps against respiratory and fungal infections; used in a steam treatment to inhale for bronchitis, coughs, congestion, and excess mucous; helps with menstrual delay, uterine contractions, venereal warts, and gonorrhea; used to treat kidney and urinary tract infections; soothes headaches; helps with rheumatism; used to treat arthritis; treats inflammation of the skin and joints, and used as a bath soak, poultice, or a salve to help with skin conditions such as eczema, dermatitis, psoriasis, dandruff, acne, and oily skin; is a diuretic; stimulates circulation.

Contraindications: Do not use if pregnant or breastfeeding.

Magical Rootwork Elements: Used during ancestor reverence and healing. I use it as an incense to call the ancestors into a sacred space or to help bring their energy to clear out negative energy.

Chasteberry or Vitex (*Vitex agnus-castus*)

Traditional Uses: Regulates female hormones; helps with premenstrual syndrome (PMS) and menopause; balances reproductive hormones.

Contraindications: May reduce the effectiveness of hormonal birth control.

Magical Rootwork Elements: Used with women for energetic womb healing, fertility, and love magic.

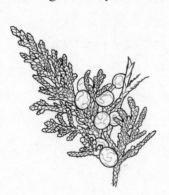

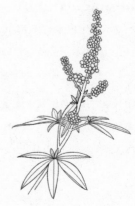

Cedar   Chasteberry or Vitex

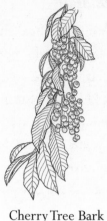

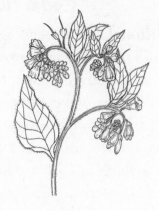

Cherry Tree Bark   Comfrey

Cherry Tree Bark (*Prunus avium* or *Prunus serotina*)

Traditional Uses: Aids digestion; alleviates colds, coughs, respiratory ailments, and congestion.

Contraindications: A strong medicine; use in small doses.

Magical Rootwork Elements: Used in matters of the heart to bring luck and attraction.

Comfrey (*Symphytum officinale*)

Traditional Uses: Helps heal injuries by stimulating cell growth; used externally in compresses, poultices, washes, and salves.

Contraindications: Safe for topical use; avoid internal use during pregnancy, breastfeeding, when cancer or tumors are present, or when there is a history of liver problems. The herbalist community is having a debate about the safety of comfrey's internal use, especially long term.

Magical Rootwork Elements: This plant is beautiful! I use it in spiritual baths to heal energetic wounds (such as heartbreak, grief, and so on), especially with the sacred heart space. Promotes safety while traveling and a peaceful home.

Corn Silk (*Stigma maydis*)

Traditional Uses: Is a diuretic; relieves inflammation of kidneys and urinary tract conditions; used for anti-bedwetting; helps with cystitis; helps with gout.

Contraindications: As a diuretic, it can affect medication levels.

Magical Rootwork Elements: Used for good luck, protection, increasing psychic visions, drawing in love, fertility spells, abundance, and attracting money.

Cotton Root (*Gossypium herbaceum*)

Traditional Uses: Emmenagogue (helps promote the flow of menstrual blood and release congestion in the pelvis); assists in easing menstrual cramping and helps ease excessive bleeding; induces labor and aids labor contractions. The chewed bark and tea were used by enslaved women as an abortifacient (to cause abortion).

Contraindications: Avoid during pregnancy. Can cause uterine contractions and be a natural abortifacient.

Magical Rootwork Elements: This powerful plant tells many stories about our people. It was one of the plants that helped perpetuate enslavement (in the cotton industry of the South). It was also the plant that helped liberate women by giving them control over their bodies by choosing to be pregnant or not.

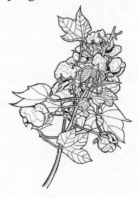

Cotton Root

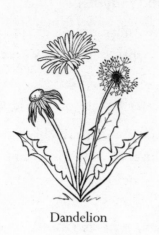 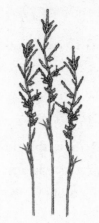

Dandelion   Devil's Shoestring

Dandelion *(Taraxacum officinale)*

Traditional Uses: Supports the liver, gallbladder, and kidney; addresses anemia by being rich in iron and gently boosting the production of red blood cells in the body; is a tonic (formula for a specific action for overall wellness), diuretic, and laxative; topically the white liquid is good for treating warts.

Contraindications: May cause an allergic skin reaction in some people. As a diuretic, it can affect medication levels.

Magical Rootwork Elements: I love this plant for self-transformation work. From root to flower, she holds deep medicine. The dandelion teaches us that even in our darkest times, medicine like the root is still happening. And like the leaf and the flower that emerge from that root, we, too, can grow into greatness. This plant grants wishes.

Devil's Shoestring *(Viburnum alnifolium)* (also called cramp bark)

Traditional Uses: An antispasmodic that relieves menstrual cramps; prevents miscarriages; and supports women's health.

Contraindications: Not for use during pregnancy or lactation.

Magical Rootwork Elements: Used for protection; worn in a gris-gris bag for gambling or when searching for a job to bring luck.

Elder/Elderberry (*Sambucus canadensis*)

Traditional Uses: Builds immunity; purifies blood; reduces inflammation; shortens duration of the flu; soothes mucous membranes and skin sores; acts as a laxative and tonic.

Contraindications: The bark, stem, and roots are mildly toxic, and can cause nausea and diarrhea. Flowers and berries should be dried, and fresh berries should be boiled for three minutes before preserving.

Magical Rootwork Elements: Offers protection and good luck.

Eucalyptus (*Eucalyptus globulus*)

Traditional Uses: It may act as an expectorant for damp coughs or asthma, lingering bronchitis, and some cases of chronic obstructive pulmonary disease (COPD). The oil can be diffused and inhaled and applied topically in a salve or oil infusion as an analgesic for arthritis. The plant is also used in steam-inhalation treatments or infused into an oil for insect repellent; eases arthritis and sore joints.

Contraindications: Use essential oil with caution in children under the age of four due to possible neurotoxicity.

Magical Rootwork Elements: Used daily in Haiti as an incense to clear negative energies. I use it in bundles and powder form. It helped

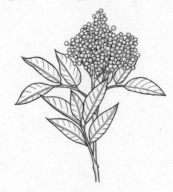

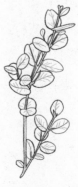

Elder/Elderberry   Eucalyptus

me put the sage wand down, since sage is endangered due to overuse, learning other plants to use for this purpose helped me expand my knowledge of what to use for certain situations. I also will use it in spiritual baths to move negative energies in the body.

Goldenrod (*Solidago virgaurea*)

Traditional Uses: Is a diuretic for urinary tract problems and obstructions, kidney stones; supports healthy liver function; helps reduce inflammation in the body; used topically for pain related to arthritis; used to treat hay fever, allergies, upper respiratory infections, yeast infections, and muscle soreness; treats colds, flu, and coughs.

Contraindications: Not for use for edema from kidney failure.

Magical Rootwork Elements: I love to use this herb in my abundance ceremonies as an offering and in my spiritual baths.

Hawthorn Berry (*Crataegus oxyacantha*)

Traditional Uses: Builds the heart and improves heart muscle tone, oxygen uptake, and circulation; dilates blood vessels in the body's extremities; helps general cardiac function.

Contraindications: Not for use for those who are pregnant or have heart conditions or hypersensitivity to Crataegus products.

Magical Rootwork Elements: Hawthorn berry is beautiful, energetic, heart-healing medicine and a must for broken hearts that need

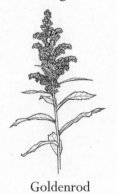

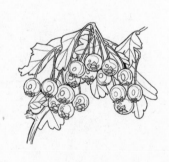

Goldenrod   Hawthorn Berry

AFRICAN AMERICAN HERBALISM

that grandmother's love energy to help heal them. Use it for protection, fertility, and happiness.

Horehound (*Marrubium vulgare*)

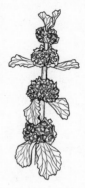

Traditional Uses: Alleviates coughs, congestion, wheezing, and difficulty breathing; stimulates digestion.

Contraindications: Use with caution during pregnancy.

Magical Rootwork Elements: Aids in protection and exorcism.

Horehound

Horny Goat Weed (*Epimedium grandiflorum*)

Traditional Uses: Alleviates sexual dysfunction, fatigue, and arthritis; builds bone mass.

Contraindications: High doses may result in difficulty breathing, dizziness, vomiting, thirst, and dry mouth.

Magical Rootwork Elements: When you want that mojo going, add this into your bath or tea before making love. It is good for calling passion into your life.

Jerusalem Weed (*Chenopodium ambrosioides*) (also known as Jerusalem oak)

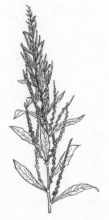

Traditional Uses: Used as a wash to treat skin fungi such as ringworm or athlete's foot; expels intestinal worms; alleviates digestive disorders, coughs, colds, congestion, diarrhea, fevers, gout, and cramps.

Contraindications: Oil extracted from the weed and seed can be highly toxic.

Jerusalem Weed

Magical Rootwork Elements: None.

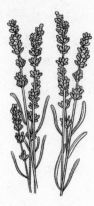
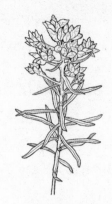

Lavender   Life Everlasting "Rabbit Tobacco"

Lavender (*Lavendula angustifolia, formerly L. officinalis*)

Traditional Uses: Is a nervine and relaxer; eases tension and anxiety; is a mood enhancer, mild antidepressant, and mild analgesic; essential oil is antifungal and good for burns; used topically in infused oils and skin care products, teas, and tinctures.

Contraindications: None known.

Magical Rootwork Elements: A wise native woman once taught me that lavender teaches us that healing does not have to be hard. Lavender gives us grace during moments of healing and transformation. I add a little lavender in every spiritual bath and burn it as an incense. We all need more grace in our lives.

Life Everlasting "Rabbit Tobacco"
(*Gnaphalium obtusifolium*)

Traditional Uses: Eases the issues associated with asthma, bronchitis, coughs, colds, and sinusitis; used as a digestive aid. The elders say, "When this plant is in your life, sickness rarely comes." That is why they named it "life everlasting." Used in smoking blends and teas, and or as a tincture.

AFRICAN AMERICAN HERBALISM

Contraindications: None known when used properly.

Magical Rootwork Elements: Used for longevity, health, and healing spells, as well as keeping sickness out of the home.

Mullein *(Verbascum thapsus)*

Traditional Uses: As an expectorant, mullein helps respiratory issues, coughs, colds, pain, rashes, earaches, lower back pain, and inflammation. Used in teas and smoking blends.

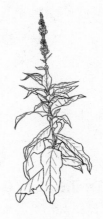

Contraindications: The leaves contain the chemical compound coumarin, and those taking blood thinners should exercise great caution when using any product containing mullein. Use of the younger inner leaves of the plant is recommended, as the larger outer leaves may cause nightmares.

Mullein

Magical Rootwork Elements: Often used as a substitute for graveyard dirt to add extra juju into your magic; used for courage, protection, and love drawing; wards off nightmares and negativity; helps with divination.

Mustard *(Brassica juncea)*

Traditional Uses: Relieves chest congestion and coughs due to flu, bronchitis, and pneumonia; expels mucus; is anti-inflammatory; alleviates joint pain, headaches, toothaches, and neuralgia; stimulates and increases blood circulation and dilation of capillaries.

Contraindications: Mustard plasters may easily irritate the skin if they are made too strong.

Magical Rootwork Elements: Used in its various forms for anything from good luck to money drawing to confusing enemies; removes hexes.

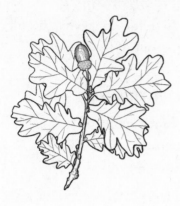

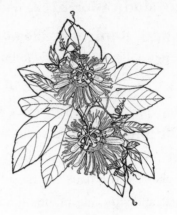

Oak Tree Bark   Passionflower/Maypop

Oak Tree Bark (*Quercus robur*)

Traditional Uses: Reduces swelling and inflammation; used as a treatment for dental conditions such as tooth decay and gum disease; aids digestion; used as a treatment for ulcers, spleen, and gallbladder problems; reduces size of kidney stones; prevents infections; and used as a skin wash to treat minor cuts, burns, insect bites, and other skin irritations.

Contraindications: May cause upset stomach and skin irritations.

Magical Rootwork Elements: None.

Passionflower/Maypop (*Passiflora incarnata*)

Traditional Uses: Is an antispasmodic, nervine, sleep aid, and nonnarcotic pain reliever for fever; quiets the mind. Used as tea and/or as a tincture.

Contraindications: No known ones.

Magical Rootwork Elements: Helps with popularity; brings peace into situations.

Pine (White) (*Pinus strobus*)

Traditional Uses: Boosts immune system and helps prevent coughs and colds, sore throat, bronchitis, kidneys; aids in chest colds, especially helping rid the body of thick green mucus. Pine gum is good for healing wounds, drawing out pus and splinters. Pine pollen strengthens muscles and tendons and helps with tissue repair. It also contains testosterone. Used in teas and infused oils, and as a tincture. Cones, needles, sap, and bark are used.

Contraindications: Should be avoided by those who are pregnant or breast feeding, children under six years old, and those with iron deficiency anemia; can cause kidney irritation with long-term use in strong doses or with sensitive individuals. A pine plaster can raise a blister.

Magical Rootwork Elements: Used for healing intergenerational trauma and honoring the ancestors.

Poke Root (*Phytolacca decandra*)

Traditional Use: Helps with lymph congestion. The elders say it is used to "clean you out" by purging the intestinal system; aids in weight loss; treats arthritis; used as a blood purifier. The root, leaf (poke salat, a salad dish), and berry are used. Used as a salve or oil to treat boils, rashes, bites, and other wounds.

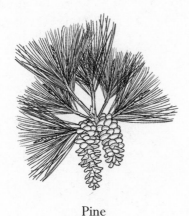

Pine

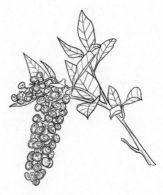

Poke Root

Contraindications: Use with extreme caution under medical supervision! Consuming large amounts can be toxic. The seeds are mildly toxic if chewed or crushed. The root is extremely toxic without proper preparation.

Magical Rootwork Elements: Used to move things quicker. I used it to push things out of my life that no longer served me.

Sage *(Salvia officinalis)*

Traditional Uses: Is an a astringent, tonic, hair wash, and nervine; helps with sleep, cramps, and colds; is a diaphoretic (increases perspiration).

Contraindications: Exercise caution when pregnant, and do not use in early pregnancy.

Magical Rootwork Elements: Used for protection and to bring wisdom and clarity.

Sarsaparilla *(Smilax pumila)*

Traditional Uses: The tea was drunk as a blood purifier; may help with menstrual disorders and menopause; may regulate hormone levels; used for psoriasis, arthritis, coughs, and colds; is a general healer and anti-inflammatory; may aid those with issues with gout and rheumatism.

Contraindications: Avoid if you have kidney problems.

Magical Rootwork Elements: Helps draw luck, love, and money.

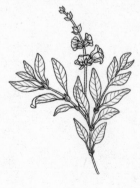

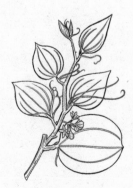

Sage   Sarsaparilla

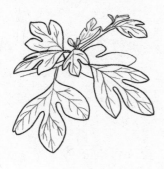

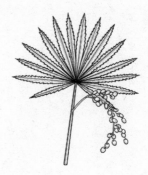

Sassafras   Saw Palmetto

Sassafras (*Sassafras albidum*)

Traditional Uses: Commonly used for colds and as a tonic during the change of the season to prevent illness; used as a hair wash; fights against lice; is a blood purifier and antiviral; soothes sore eyes; helps to treat shingles, chicken pox, and herpes.

Contraindications: None with normal usage, but sassafras contains the chemical compound safrole, which has been linked to cancer in lab rats.

Magical Rootwork Elements: Helpful for money drawing, business success, health, and healing.

Saw Palmetto (*Sabal serrulate*)

Traditional Uses: Used for prostate enlargement and urinary problems in men; is a general tonic for elderly men and assists other issues associated with aging; aids digestion and fights weight gain.

Contraindications: Avoid during pregnancy and breastfeeding.

Magical Rootwork Elements: None.

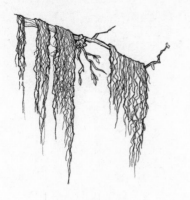

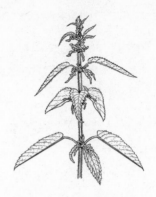

Spanish Moss   Nettles (Stinging)

Spanish Moss (*Tillandsia usneoides*)

Traditional Uses: Treats diabetes; it may regulate glucose levels; soothes fevers, skin rashes, and irritations.

Contraindications: None.

Magical Rootwork Elements: Provides protection for self and home, and energetic cleaning of the body.

Nettles (Stinging) (*Urtica dioica*)

Traditional Uses: Builds healthy blood, joints, and bones; high iron content helps with anemia, low blood pressure; is an anti-inflammatory; eases respiratory issues and allergies. Nettle seeds can slow, halt, or even partially reverse progressive renal failure.

Contraindications: The fresh plant can be painful to the touch and cause skin irritation.

Magical Rootwork Elements: Provides protection from negative forces.

Tobacco (*Nicotiana tabacum*)

Traditional Uses: Soothes bee stings, insect bites, snakebites, earaches, and skin wounds; acts as an antiseptic; alleviates constipation and ulcers; expels intestinal worms.

Contraindications: No known ones for topical use. May cause dizziness or vomiting for internal use (use with caution and guidance). Choose only pure tobacco for internal use.

Magical Rootwork Elements: A very sacred ceremonial plant to many indigenous cultures, tobacco was used to help connect to the spirit world; it is also used as an offering or to show gratitude, or to purify the body from illness or trauma. The smoke is used to bless other medicines or tools for healing practices.

Wormwood (*Artemisia absinthium*)

Traditional Uses: Antiparasitic—expels tapeworms and other internal parasites; stimulates digestion and appetite.

Contraindications: A very strong, potentially toxic herb. Not recommended for use by pregnant and nursing women; recommended for short-term use.

Magical Rootwork Elements: Helps with developing psychic powers and protection from accidents; calls in spirits to help.

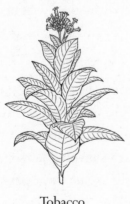

Tobacco

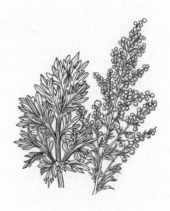

Wormwood

CHAPTER 4

SPIRITUAL BATHING WITH THE ELEMENTS

In all my travels as a medicine woman and herbalist, I have witnessed plants used in many powerful ceremonies for healing, protection, purification, abundance, and personal transformation. Early in my journey, I learned about the practice of spiritual bathing; I have seen and experienced this ritual having one of the biggest effects on a person's spiritual well-being.

In a church downriver from my childhood home, I witnessed baptisms in pools at church as well as the river, where the power of water and prayers combined with the "laying on of the hands" (similar to reiki or energy work) would have people looking new and freer. As a young child I would think to myself, "I am going to do *that* when I am older." Those moments inspired my journey to see what "that" was and how I could discover ways to make people feel better and assist them on their own journeys.

Spiritual bathing is using plants in their metaphysical and medicinal form to facilitate healing on both an energetic and physical level. Also, this bathing uses the elements of fire, water, earth, sound, air (using incense), or nature to facilitate healing. It can involve personal ceremonies to be used on ourselves, to spiritually cleanse our pets, and to protect our homes as well. Also, spiritual bathing is related to an ancient technique—still used today—of rolling an egg all over the body. Many African cultures embrace this practice to remove negative energies and help infertility issues, as well as heal women in the area of the womb.

I have rarely seen spiritual bathing in Western versions of herbalism and healing arts. To me, this absence means missing out on half of the power of the plants and a beautiful gateway to healing the soul and energetic body.

Many indigenous cultures understand that to fully allow the plants to heal all levels of the mind, body, and spirit, you have to invoke and evoke their power in all ways. I have seen and experienced firsthand the power of plants to move one beyond grief, reveal things that are needed, and assist in healing the body.

Over the course of twenty-five years, I have heard many personal stories of illness and have connected those illnesses to an emotional or energetic root. Hearing these stories inspired me to dig deeper into creating treatment protocols and approach each person's unique situation so I could understand the holistic synergy of body, mind, and spirit.

Think about it—we take herbs, eat well, and exercise to support the body. We meditate, see our therapist (maybe), and take herbs to help the mind. But how do we feed and heal the spirit? Indigenous practitioners have always known that the spirit is one of the most important parts to healing and would prepare many kinds of remedies to address it, along with the body. Baths, along with a prayer, symbols, or a mantra, would be used throughout the healing process. This way of healing can give you a personal role in your own journey to wellness.

From birth to death, spiritual bathing ceremonies are very important in African American culture. Elements such as incense, sacred water, decocted plants (plants cooked down in the process of extracting the essence or medicine of herbs), sound, and even "forest bathing" are used to bring balance. There are baths to attract love, remove sickness, help with grief, bring abundance, enhance fertility, accomplish purification, and facilitate breakups and divorce to cut cords of past relationship. As you can see, there is a bath for pretty much everything. I have always used baths in my own personal and professional practice. I find a bath to be one of the most powerful modalities for times of transition, healing, and transformation.

Using the Elements for Spiritual Baths

Forest Bathing

The importance of sound as a healing modality has been passed down from the ancient Egyptians and woven into newer ways. I have always used the practice of infusing prayers and songs into my herbal medicines. I recommend my clients to do the same when taking the medicine. Create a playlist that inspires different emotions or sing whatever makes your spirit happy. In her business Vibration of Grace, one of my colleagues and beloved friends, sound healer Gina Breedlove, suggests saying your own name to yourself to call back your power.

Living legacy Rickie Byars is a sound healer, music alchemist, fellow North Carolina native, music director, and powerhouse that inspired many at Agape International Spiritual Center. She reminds us to speak the language of Spirit and reminds us of the power of song. When you experience one of her devotional musical concerts, you are reminded that simply placing your hand on your heart and listening to the right kind of music can send a transformational vibration that calls you back home to yourself. When Byars went through a divorce, I asked her what one practice grounds her quickly in her times of transition. This is what she told me.

As a child, she would lean up against a pine tree in her front yard, and she would dream. The trees have always brought her comfort in times of change. Now, as an adult, while creating her new life and new vision for her work, she has come back to this practice to realign herself in her garden. "I lay my spine against the pine tree at my home and feel it align me … not only my physical body but my spirit."

The pine is a sacred tree used to heal intergenerational and ancestral trauma. It is not an accident that the Christmas tree is a pine. We all need a little help with all the emotions of the holidays.

We have all heard of the term "tree hugger." There is, however, a science behind forest bathing, or being in nature with the trees. It leads to a substantial increase in oxytocin, which is the hormone your body produces during moments of emotional bonding. With social distancing during the pandemic, imagine how this practice could help so many people. Trees produce oxygen, which is the life force. The color green (a heart chakra color) is also said to lower systolic blood pressure and keep the heart rate more balanced.

Many African cultures have always had a deep connection to the trees and their healing properties. A wide range of African ceremonies and rituals are centered on trees, consisting of activities like bathing in the forest atmosphere or taking in the forest through the senses. A mindfulness practice can begin with immersing in the sounds of nature so you can hear yourself and your ancestors more clearly.

Byars and I also talked about using the elements of sound and song to deepen this forest-bathing experience as it connects to Africa. Byars explained that "sound recalibrates the body and helps alter our DNA; it is the original language of the universe."

We spoke of African cultures in which a woman wanting to have a child would go into the woods to listen for the song of the child to come. That song would be sung throughout the woman's life in times when she needed strength from the village and to remember who she was. Byars also talked about the power of a song or personal mantra to ignite the fire of change and to reclaim your power. May you speak sweetness to yourself and find a soul song.

Healing Power of Water

Water is such a sacred tool for healing and one of our most valuable resources for life. As previously mentioned, water can carry vibrations that we can use in many aspects of our life. Water is such an important part in spiritual bathing because it releases and amplifies plant energies in the healing and purification process. Even if you do not use plants, you can still benefit from using the sound of your voice and a prayer to create a simple spiritual bath for yourself. From drinking a glass of water to taking a shower, you can infuse deep healing into your every-day activities.

Florida Water

Florida water is an old-time, hidden-in-plain-sight ceremonial potion. This remedy is used in both spiritual ceremonies and baths. Named after the healing springs in Florida that, according to folklore, were known as the fountain of youth, Florida water was widely adapted for use in the hoodoo (see page 140), voodoo, and Santeria cultures. It is used throughout the Caribbean and US, and you can buy it at many botanicas.

Since much of our magic was hidden in plain sight due to laws and restrictions forbidding African Americans from practicing our traditions, Florida water resembles a simple cologne sold in many drugstores. This enabled our people to practice unbeknownst to others who might have reported them for their spiritual traditions.

I have been to many ceremonies that use this water, most recently at the Spiritualist Church of New Orleans. I use it in my personal practices as well. I call myself a connoisseur of Florida water because I love to collect homemade versions from different cultures and practitioners. They differ depending on what plants are used and the intent of the formula, as well as the smell. Florida water is used to anoint and cleanse anything, including your altar's objects and your body. Altars can be utilized and customized for various reasons. They can be used to honor your ancestors or specific religious deities, as places to meditate or celebrate specific holidays, for protection of your home/self, and many other purposes. You can also energetically cleanse your home by adding Florida water to your floor washes, and you can wipe down doors and windows to remove negative energies. Murray & Lanman Florida water was one of the first brands on the market in the 1800s and is the go-to brand for most people. Here is a recipe to make your own that uses only botanicals. Many people add essential oils as a final step. I love to collect my citrus peels and use them after I eat the fruits. These recipes are personal, so follow your own intuition and use what you are drawn to.

peel of 3 lemons

peel of 3 limes

peel of 3 oranges

handful fresh basil (I love to add tulsi, or holy basil)

3 or 4 springs fresh rosemary

9 bay leaves

handful dried jasmine

3 to 6 cinnamon sticks

9 or more cloves

handful mugwort

7 or so juniper berries

2 handfuls roses

full stick of palo santo wood

3 star anise pods

handful calendula

handful five finger grass (to add in more money manifesting power)

enough vodka to finish covering plant material (at least 100 proof; you also can use Everclear or overproof rum)

1 (8-ounce) bottle of your favorite rose water

~~~~~~~~~~

1. Begin with an ancestor prayer and sacred incense to clear the air. Also play music to fit the mood you want to invoke with this potion.

2. With focused intent and prayers, place all your botanical ingredients (those ingredients that precede the vodka) into a glass container large enough to fit everything.

3. Cover with vodka (or rum, if using) until it is at least 1 inch above the materials.

4. Add in the rose water.

5. Allow the mixture to sit for three moon cycles or longer, shaking it up weekly to add your energy and more prayers (if you choose the new moon or full moon, wait till the moon comes around three times). You also can let it sit for a shorter time, following your intuition.

6. If desired, add crystals like citrine (for money), rose quartz (for love, especially self-love), or any stone you are drawn to. I put them near the mixture or on top of it.

7. Write a prayer or mantra and place it under the container to add a more focused intent while it is brewing.

How to Come into Full Bloom

To make a flower bath, just add flowers, water, earth, prayer, salt, and the elemental force of nature, and you have the recipe to help heal the soul. Jacquelin Guiteau, one of the teachers I have been blessed to study with, taught me the importance of flower baths according to his tradition. "Flowers and flower essences heal the psychic and emotional body"—this is a major part of Guiteau's work and teachings.

A spiritual teacher and herbalist for twenty years, Guiteau's herbalism journey began in his native Haiti, where the veil of the spiritual world is thin. In class and his book *The Breath of the Divine*, he spoke of seeing his mother waking up every day to burn eucalyptus, using the smoke or the element of air as a "spiritual bath" to clear the energy in the home. This practice can also be used on the body with so many different plants.[27]

He has studied Western and Eastern mysticism extensively since the age of fourteen and spent three years in India studying in a Buddhist monastery. He always says healing should always come with the secret ingredient … love.

During our time together we made four baths. Three were made of flowers: a pink one for the heart and love; yellow calendula for spreading abundance on all levels (joy, money, happiness) equally through life; and white flowers for purifying. The fourth bath was a combination of mint, rosemary, and basil, and was used first to open the way for the other ones to work.

Each bath had to be made outside in the full sun for hours, never letting the shadow hit them during the process. These types of baths are not for the faint of heart and are integral to a ceremony to facilitate healing. Like most traditional baths, they are cold and the components are rigorously scrubbed and slapped all over the body. Doing this moves the energy and truly gets the plant medicine *in* and whatever negative or blocked energy that is holding you back *out*. Cold baths are used in many different cultures to extract negative energies.

In Guiteau's tradition, you begin with the mint, basil, and rosemary bath first to help move the blockages to begin the purification. You then follow with the flower bath to heal and bring about your intent of the session. We have so much to learn from Haiti's connection to the plants and the spiritual world.

---

27 Let us move away from the overuse of sage, which has become so widely used that it is becoming endangered. I hope this chapter gives many people a reason to put down the sage bundles and pick up more plants and resins to help facilitate a more sustainable love for the plants and more respect for the indigenous people's medicine.

When I create a bath, the plants tell a story of what needs to happen to facilitate the healing process. Some baths are done once, some three times, and some for seven days. Your spiritual healer can best determine what process you need, but feel free to use your own intuition.

I am always making formulas not only for my clients, but also for my own personal transformation and healing. We all get lost at times in the sentiment "what am I really doing on this planet?" And in the work I do with grief and trauma, I also have to constantly practice finding ways to move those emotions energetically from my body, mind, and spirit. We all have also had relationships that have broken us and often realize we are not in spaces that truly feed our soul. I find this practice truly gives us the ceremonies to move forward, break ties, and help deal with the waves of grief that come over us. I will share a personal story where this modality was truly beneficial to me, along with some client profiles and recipes.

I recently used the knowledge of spiritual bathing in my personal practice at a critical time of transition and heartbreak. This past year of the pandemic has taught us many things; we had to let go of so much we thought we could not live without. It made us pull closer together or fall further apart as I have seen in some circles of modern herbalism.

I found I was somewhere in the middle, so I turned to the power inspired by Guiteau and a traditional recipe for a "white spiritual bath" that helped with depression, post-traumatic stress disorder (PTSD), anxiety, and purification, and it balanced my emotions. This bath is said to cool these energies. I used it to help pull me through to what the spirit had in store for me ... to purify myself ... to get out of my way. I was ready to release whatever had me energetically stuck.

I also wanted to focus more clearly and use this time to "feed my Ori" or head energy. Ori, literally meaning "head," refers to one's spiritual intuition and destiny. It is human consciousness embedded in the human essence and therefore is often referred to as an orisha in itself. It is also one of the major reasons why we as a people do not like anyone touching our hair. The head is of huge significant spiritual importance to our entire being. It is also a reason that some wear head wraps to protect the energy of the head.

When we are children, people tell us what they think we should do, act like, or be. As we grow older, we go through so much trauma and stress in our lives, this Ori energy is often depleted. We lose focus, get disenchanted and confused, lose trust in our own voice—or we cannot hear our sacred purpose as clearly any more. Sometimes we never have. The old ways had ceremonies for this. Also the village would have known what your purpose was before you came, and everyone would be there to support you in that journey. What if life was still like that? How beautiful would that be?

At the beginning of the pandemic, I decided to commit to a seven-day spiritual bath. I felt something was off in my life, so I set out to wander through my yard apothecary to find the stories and medicine that Mother Nature had for me. So much of what we need is right outside our door. I love to see where my spirit leads me; then I look up the spiritual meaning of the plants. I will always be a student of the plants.

Spring means flowers early in the South; I met a new flower friend I had growing next door that I never noticed. Mock orange flower helps when you are stuck in old emotional patterns often relating to anger, fear, and low self-esteem; it offers the power to endure difficult situation. I sat with her and prayed, and through plant spirit meditation, she gifted me with the knowledge of her medicine to add to the recipe. I am always in awe of how the right plant will show up when you need it!

I gathered yarrow used in healing the wounded healer; it had abnormally grown earlier in the season.

Honeysuckle had shown herself early as well; her energy helps you walk in your own power and know your own worth.

Wisteria always brings me joy; her energy inspires us to climb higher to expand our creativity, and she speaks of lost love and of the ability for the heart to endure in spite of loss.

I added some white dogwood flowers, which help to purify and protect. They symbolize sacrifice, the ones we have made and will make to nourish our gifts. White dogwood also helps you stand fully in your personal power.

I also chose holy basil to align the crown chakra and to move any negative energies and traumas, as her medicine is great for PTSD.

I chose lavender to show me that healing does not have to be difficult and to allow grace into my soul.

I added mimosa leaf and dried flower for moving deep grief, mugwort to swiftly move any stagnant energy, comfrey to heal my heart wounds, and roses for heart healing and protection. A few drops of poke root tincture in the concoction pushed it all through (I was not playing).

Finally, I added okra pods and okra flower essence I had made the previous year. Okra helps move deep stagnant energy in the lower chakra. To that I added a can of coconut milk (you could also use regular cow milk).

I was ready. I lit my candles, put my crystals in the water, and prayed. After the first bath, my love of seven years said they needed space and had begun a life outside us. I was heartbroken and taken off axis. I thought, "Really spirit, this is DAY ONE?! Where will I live? I am not even working. The world is upside down and the baby girl in me is here again, repeating a story of abandonment." In tears and truly heartbroken, I dragged myself to that tub every day for seven days. I sang the songs and chanted deep healing words into my heart. Then, by day three, on the new moon, the tsunamis started hitting less hard, and I could begin to see the forest for the trees. I could breathe and started the path to loving myself back to center. Once again, I turned to the plants, my ancestors, the spirit, and my tribe. I also began holding space for myself as a deeper practice. We as healers, parents, and humans often forget the importance of this because by constantly helping heal others, we forget ourselves.

Going through this divorce and having to leave an entire life during a pandemic has been one of the craziest adventures of my life. I have had wild adventures, such as running with elephants, but I am a living testament to how the energetic power of the plants can help manifest and heal under the most difficult situations.

A year later, the free-spirited, adventure-seeking, barefoot girl who lives big is seeing love come flowing back from all areas of her life. I have not seen her in a very long time. Sometimes we do not realize how much of ourselves we lose trying to love and support someone else. Love may not at all look like what I thought it would, but the plants have shown me it is so much bigger than I could imagine. My life has opened up so much, and the people I have met along the way have been so beautiful! It has been possible using the main ingredient for alchemy … love.

Elemental Bathing Recipes and Ceremonies

FOREST BATHING USING SOUND

1. Find your favorite space in the forest.
2. Sit with your back against a tree and begin taking deep belly breaths.

3. When your mind begins to settle, allow the sounds of the forest to come in; notice the smells, and how the wind, the earth beneath you, and the tree feel.

4. Place your hand on your heart and sing the favorite song of your soul; chant "I AM" or simply scream to release.

5. Gently rise and hug the tree, thanking it for the medicine while slowly walking away.

ANCESTOR CONNECTION BATH

Bring the forest to your bathtub. This is used for grounding, ancestor connection, and mental clarity. This bath experience pairs well with pine, and peppermint tea to sip. Add in skullcap or passion flower to the tea for extra chill.

medium-size pot of water

¼ cup lavender buds

1 cup fresh pine needles, plus more for incense

1 cup fresh cedar leaves

1 teaspoon clay or fresh earth (dirt)

1 to 2 cups Epsom salts or sea salt

1 dropper St. John's wort extract or 5 drops of the essential oil (optional)

4 to 6 tablespoons Babassu oil or another tree-based oil

3 tablespoons cedar wood powder

palo santo wood (optional)

1. Bring the water to a boil and turn off the heat.

2. Add the lavender buds, fresh pine needles, and fresh cedar leaves.

3. Cover and let steep for 45 minutes to 2 hours.

4. Drain and add to bathwater.

5. To the bathwater, add the clay or mud, the Epsom or sea salt, and the St. John's wort or essential oil. Add the bath oil, if using. Burn the pine needles, cedar wood powder, or palo santo wood as an incense to add to the element of air. You can also light a candle to bring in the element of fire to your spiritual bath process.

TIPS

If you do not have the space or find it difficult to find the time, you can also turn this or any spiritual bath into a spiritual bath salt scrub by not boiling the plants but putting them into a coffee grinder or blender until they are a fine powder. Then add that to 2 cups of fine salt. Top it off with your favorite oil (I love to use my infused medicinal oils). Mix well and place into a jar for later use. If made with fresh herbs, this will keep for 6 months; with dried herbs or just essential oils, it will keep for 1 year.

You can also add essential oils like these to complement and give the bath more fragrance:

* Essential oils: combination of two or three (optional), using 3 to 4 drops
* Cedar (honor the ancestors and purify the spirit)
* Pine (helps heal family traumas)
* Atlas cedarwood
* Palo santo
* Grapefruit (for mental elevation)
* Lavender (for relaxation)

FULL BLOOM SPIRIT RECIPE

This is inspired by a variation of the traditional white bath recipe, intended to cleanse the aura of negative energy.

mugwort (to move stagnant energy in the body)

holy basil (to help with trauma)

comfrey (to heal cuts and pain physically or energetically)

lavender (to give peace and grace to the healing process)

yarrow (to help energetically to heal the wounded healer)

6 okra pods or a full dropper okra flower essence (optional; to help clear the body of negative energy)

fresh white flowers

½ to 1 (13.5-ounce) can coconut, goat, or cow milk

1. Boil water in a medium pot, turn off the burner, and place a small handful of each herb in the pot.

2. Allow it to infuse for 45 minutes to 2 hours. Use for 3 to 7 days.

FEED YOUR ORI— A HEAD WASH FOR CLARITY

Have you ever asked yourself "Why am I here?" Sometimes we need clarity in a situation or to bring ourselves into alignment with our true purpose. Many African spiritual traditions hold the belief that we come into this world knowing our true purpose. Then, other people start clouding our memory with what they believe we should do and, we get off track. This head wash is for nourishing or feeding the Ori, purifying your spiritual connection, bringing clarity, and helping you start to align with your true purpose.

gingko (used for centuries as "brain food"; teaches us we can stand the test of time and increases energy to the brain)

peppermint (clears and cleanses the mind; helps with focus)

rosemary (increases focus)

garden basil or tulsi (holy basil; used for psychic or spiritual enhancement, purifying negative energies)

lavender (to add grace and ease in your alignment)

white flowers (to purify the energetic body and mind)

3 splashes Florida water

½ (13.5-ounce) can coconut milk

1. Boil a medium pot of water, turn off the burner, and place a small handful of each herb or a combination of a few of these herbs into the pot and cover.

2. Add in 3 splashes of Florida water and half a can of the coconut milk before using.

3. Strain and take into the shower or bath with you. Pour it over your head, pausing in between pours to massage into scalp. Do not rinse. Cover your head for sleeping. This can be divided into 3 head washes and done 3 days in a row for maximum benefits.

MONEY-DRAWING AND ABUNDANCE BATH

Last year, I had to manifest money fast to be able to quickly leave the home I had once shared, to provide financial security for myself, and to continue my work for my community. Daily prayers down by the river and a series of abundance baths brought in money and kept me with enough of it to begin to make a good life for myself.

We all follow the old folk saying about eating collard greens for the New Year—eating them will bring financial prosperity. Even if you do not believe in folklore, no one from the South is going to miss eating them on that day. I use them in my apothecary for my money root-work with baths or with candle magic. Also, as I eat any greens, I think money flows to me easily. This bath is most powerful around the new moon. When possible, I love to use fresh water from rivers or springs for this one.

enough water to fill a medium or large pot

handful bay leaves (used to purify or call in your heart's desire)

handful goldenrod leaves and flowers (used to purify or call in your heart's desire)

handful collard greens, or you can eat a bowl of them after your bath (brings in abundance)

handful calendula (brings abundance on all levels—joy, love, and money—and keeps it flowing)

small handful lavender (so money comes with ease and grace)

3 splashes Florida water

8 ounces coconut or cow's milk (optional)

¼ cup honey (optional)

1. Boil a medium or large pot of water. Turn off the burner and place a small handful of each herb or a combination of a few of these herbs into the pot and cover. Let it sit for at least 45 minutes. If working with the moon or sun energy, allow it to sit overnight in the new moon light or steep all day in the sun.

2. Strain.

3. Add in 3 splashes of Florida water and 8 ounces of the coconut milk before using in the shower or bath.

4. If you use this in the shower, pour it over your head in three pours while focusing on abundance coming to you. If you are using it while bathing, add a citrine crystal along with 8 ounces of milk and ¼ cup of honey for extra magic to draw in abundance.

5. Do not rinse off the bath. Cover your head when you go to sleep or if you have to go into public.

GRIEF RELEASE BATH

Grief requires a multilayered healing process and, sometimes, we need a little help with moving our grief. This bath helps the tsunami waves of grief move with less weight.

enough water to fill a large pot

handful mimosa leaf and flower

albizia julibrissin (helps move deep grief)

handful lavender (helps bring grace into the healing process; soothes the mind)

handful rose petals (fresh or dried; helps heal the sacred heart space and provides protection during the healing process)

small handful mugwort (helps move stagnant energy in the body)

handful lemon balm (brings in sweetness, calms, and helps heal the energetic heart)

handful rue or hyssop (used to energetically purify and protect; optional)

handful comfrey (helps mend energetic wounds)

3 splashes Florida water

8 ounces coconut or cow's milk

1. Boil a large pot of water, turn off the burner, and place a small handful of each herb or a combination of a few of these herbs into the pot and cover. Let it steep for 45 minutes to 3 hours. If working with the moon energies, allow it to sit overnight in the full moon light for extra energetic release.

2. Strain the herbs out keep bathtub drain from clogging.

3. Add in 3 splashes of Florida water and 8 ounces of the coconut or cow's milk.

4. Pour mixture into your bath and soak in the power of the plants.

PURIFICATION BATH

This bath is perfect for when you feel stuck or need to feel freeier of negative energy. Use once a month during the full moon for extra release. When possible I love to collect fresh spring, river, or ocean water for this one.

enough water to fill a large pot

6 okra pods (to help purge the body of negative and stagnant energy)

handful mugwort (helps move stagnant energy in the body; optional)

handful lavender (teaches us healing does not have to be hard and soothes the mind, body, and soul)

handful hyssop (for purifying and protection; optional)

handful rue (for spiritual cleanses and protection; optional)

3 splashes Florida water

1. Fill a large pot with water that you have prayed over, asking for the healing needed. Add the okra pods and boil for 20 minutes.

2. Turn off the heat, add in the rest of the plants and flowers, as well as the Florida water, and cover the pot. Let steep for at 1 hour to overnight in the full moon light.

3. You can place a piece of black tourmaline crystal into the pot to "infuse" the energy of the crystal, or place it with you in the bathwater.

4. Strain out the plant material and just add this liquid into the bath or pour it over yourself in the shower.

TIP

Okra water is also very good for the body and has many amazing benefits due to its due mucilage properties. After boiling the okra pods in filtered drinkable water only and before adding other herbs or Florida water, remove the okra water and drink 8 ounces of the warm okra water.

TRAUMA BLEND AND PERSONAL PROTECTION BATH

I see clients for various issues. One of the hardest things that people move through is the trauma of domestic violence. This is one recipe I used with a client who came to me after an episode with their partner. If we can quickly get to people soon after these experiences, we can help move the energies trapped in the body after the trauma. These baths do not completely take away the experiences, but they work on the energetic body to help recalibrate the person to move closer to the healing process. It is also important to provide healing for the children in the home.

enough water to fill a medium to large pot

handful black or English walnuts (for cutting ties with things not serving us and for breaking bonds of relationships when a partner is ready to move forward)

handful holy basil (for PTSD)

handful lavender (for relaxation, opening the way for an easier path to healing)

handful mugwort (for moving negative and stagnant energy)

3 star anise pods (for protection)

handful roses (for self-love, healing the heart space, and protection while healing from trauma)

handful fresh white flowers (for purifying the spirit and bringing gentleness during the healing process)

1 to 2 splashes Florida water (for protecting and purifying the body, mind, and spirit)

black tourmaline crystal, rose quartz, or both (for amplifying the power of the plants; optional)

½ teaspoon fresh earth or clay (for grounding)

~~~~~~~~~

1. Fill a large pot with water that you have prayed over, asking for the healing needed. I collected fresh spring water for this one. Add the walnuts and bring the water to a boil.

2. Turn off the heat, add in the rest of the plants and flowers, as well as the Florida water, and cover the pot. I let it steep for at least an hour or sometimes overnight in the moonlight.

3. Add the small amount of fresh earth or clay, then place the black tourmaline and rose quartz crystal into the pot, if using, to "infuse" the energy of the crystal, or place them with you in the bathwater.

4. You can strain out the plant material and just add this liquid into the bath or pour it over yourself in the shower. I prefer using the traditional approach of rubbing the plant material all over your body and then pouring the bathwater over yourself.

SPIRITUAL BATH FOR CHILDREN

When my clients come to me for services that deal with grief or trauma, I always work with their children too. I think this is an area many practitioners forget about. When trauma enters the home through the parents, it affects the children, who suffer in their own way as they try to navigate through a world that now moves differently for them.

Children suffer from grief, bullying, hurt feelings, pressure to be perfect, and other traumas. The suicide rate in children is higher than ever. I had a child as a client whose father died before the child was born. He was ten and was truly missing that connection. He started acting out in ways that were not normal for him. His mother brought him to me for a session and I decided to help him deal with his grief with a spiritual bath and plant medicine suggestions. She called me two weeks later to thank me for helping her get her son back.

I was called to this bath for him and began using it for all my clients' children. I feel we need to find all the ways to hold space for them. The plants are there to assist our babies to help them in this world.

water   handful calendula
handful lemon balm   1 teaspoon holy basil or a
handful lavender   few leaves fresh basil
handful roses

~~~~~~~~~

1. Fill a medium pot with water and bring to a slight boil.

2. Turn off the stove.

3. Add in each herb and cover.

4. Allow the mixture to steep for at least 30 minutes.

5. Strain.

6. Add to bathwater or let cool to a comfortable temperature and pour it over the child.

7. After the bath, let the child sip lemon balm tea before bed.

SPIRITUAL BATHING TECHNIQUES FOR THE HOME

1. Add Florida water to your mop water or into a small bucket of water, then wipe down your windows and doors.

2. Sweeping is an ancient technique used in many countries to move negative energy outward toward the door; if you are trying to draw in money or other positive things, sweep toward the center of the room.

3. Burn herbs like eucalyptus, pine, mugwort, lavender, cedar, cypress, or your chosen favorite (I love to find other alternatives to sage) as an incense each morning and/or evening. Do this at least weekly to move

the negative energy out of the room. Open doors and windows to let out any negative energy in the house.

Sacred Skin Care

SELF-LOVE SUGAR SCRUB

Add sweetness to your soul while taking your sacred ceremonies into your bath with this amazing plant magic body scrub. For the person on the go, this is the perfect self-love spiritual bath substitute! Your resulting smooth dewy skin will also thank you.

1 tablespoon dried rose petals (to hydrate the skin, increase circulation, and bring love with protection while healing)

1 teaspoon dried calendula petals, destemmed (to soothe skin and energetically help abundance flow in all areas— love, joy, money, and so on)

1 tablespoon lavender buds (to soothe skin and bring in more peace and grace)

½ tablespoon dried hyssop (purifies the energetic body; soothing to the skin)

½ cup or more of comfrey, plantain leaf, calendula, or herbal rose-infused oil

1 tablespoon St. John's wort oil (soothes, has antibacterial properties to help with acne, aids with wound healing, and hydrates the skin; optional)

½ cup raw fine sugar (hydrating and soothing to the skin)

1 to 2 tablespoons honey (antibacterial, soothing, and hydrating; optional)

1. Place herbs into a blender or coffee grinder to just chop a little (I like to see them in my scrub).

2. Blend herbs, skin serum oil, St. John's wort oil (if using), sugar, and honey (if using), and mix well.

3. Place mixture into a labeled clean jar (I also add in a small rose quartz to charge it with the heart-healing love stone).

4. When applying this scrub to yourself in the shower, say a personal self-love mantra like: "I AM whole, I AM beautiful, I AM abundant."

SWEET GLOW HONEY LOVE FACIAL SCRUB

This hydrating soothing scrub helps leave skin smoother and brighter, and acts as a mask to leave skin glowing. It is great for all types of skin! Use more honey if needed to make the mixture smooth. Find rice flour at any Asian grocery store. To preserve your scrub, do not let any water get into the jar.

1 teaspoon dried plantain leaf (soothes skin)

1 teaspoon dried comfrey leaf (helps with wounds and sprains; leaves skin looking revived; helps with eczema, psoriasis, burns, and cuts)

1 teaspoon dried rose petals (hydrates, soothes, and helps with circulation)

1 teaspoon dried lavender (soothes skin)

1 teaspoon dried calendula (nourishes, soothes, hydrates, and brightens skin)

1 teaspoon dried holy basil (cooling and anti-inflammatory; helps with small wounds and acne; rich in vitamin C; helps boost skin cell metabolism)

1 tablespoon rice flour (for brightening)

2 to 3 tablespoons honey (hydrating; has antibacterial properties that help with acne)

1. Place all the herbs in a clean coffee grinder and grind until they are powdery fine (I like to use one coffee grinder specifically for herbs).

2. Add the rice flour and place the powdered herbs in a clean bowl.

3. Slowly pour in the honey, mixing it into the powder until the texture becomes smooth.

4. Place the mixture into a small, clean jar and label the jar.

5. Apply a small amount to your skin with a damp finger and smooth it onto your skin in an upward, circular motion.

6. Leave the scrub on for 5 to 10 minutes for a mask.

7. Rinse the scrub off well, apply rose water or toner, and apply facial oil serum.

SELF-RENEWAL PURIFYING FACIAL MASK

This powerful, rich mask soothes, purifies, plumps, hydrates, and leaves skin glowing with each use. Excellent for all skin types. Patch test on extremely sensitive skin.

1 tablespoon rolled oats or old-fashioned raw oats

½ tablespoon sea moss powder (hydrates, remineralizes, soothes, balances oil production, and gives a glow to skin)

1 tablespoon plantain leaf (soothes skin)

1 tablespoon dried rose petals (hydrates and soothes skin)

1 tablespoon dried lavender (soothes skin)

1 tablespoon Bentonite clay (removes impurities, balances oil production, adds minerals such as calcium and magnesium, helps treat acne breakouts, helps soothe poison ivy and rashes)

1 tablespoon rice flour (gently exfoliates and brightens skin)

1 to 2 tablespoons of rose water, warm water, or warm chamomile tea (hydrates, soothes, and brightens skin)

1. Place the oatmeal and herbs into a high-powered blender or coffee grinder and grind into a fine powder.

2. Place the powder into a clean bowl, add the clay and rice flour, and stir well.

3. To activate the mask, add the rose water, warm water, or warm chamomile tea for an extra-brightening effect.

4. Mix it until smooth and apply it with a mask brush or small, wide paintbrush.

5. Leave it on for 10 to 15 minutes and remove with a warm washcloth (this mask will stain a lighter-color cloth).

CHAPTER 5

"WORKING THE ROOTS"

"Working the roots" is a phrase commonly used in the South to talk about hoodoo or voodoo. Some of these were our ancient practices that were used throughout Africa and the Caribbean and brought to the Americas. They have been demonized throughout history by those who wished to erase them and to make us fear the ways our ancestors used to liberate and heal. I often use this phrase to reclaim the narrative of the rich, deep culture of medicine making and the magic of my people. I also use it in discussing the deep connection that we have to the plant work, and to talk of the ceremonial process of making medicines for health and wellness. From harvest to bottle, I find that I can make a more powerful medicine for myself, my family, and my community by mindfully participating in the entire process—from "meeting" the plant, harvesting it ethically, and creating the medicines to be administered. A simple tincture or tea can become a powerful ally to those who need it when it is made with deep love and reverence for nature and the medicine-making process. The songs we sing, the energy we carry while making the tincture or tea, our environment, and even choosing the companies we source our ingredients from are all important components.

When we work the root, we are also finding the root of an illness or problem by addressing it holistically. If we tend to the roots of not only ourselves but also the process we heal with, great things can happen.

In the old days, learning this practice was valuable because it helped preserve seasonal harvests to provide healing medicines for the upcoming seasons. These traditions of healing were passed down through the generations.

This is a guide you can use to begin to create your own apothecary; more advanced practitioners can use some of this information to add more intent into their practice.

Tincture

Tincturing involves extracting the medicinal properties of a plant by using a drinkable solvent such as vodka or other liquor. (Glycerin or even apple cider vinegar can be used in tinctures for children or for those who do not drink alcohol.) Most people used whatever was available to them. Whiskey or moonshine was the primary liquor used in the South, but now vodka or ethanol alcohol are mostly used. I suggest starting simple, and when you are comfortable and gain more knowledge, you can expand your expertise and experimentation. I like to use various liquors combined with plant materials to create medicines that honor the old ways and create blends, each of which has a different effect and flavor. My elderberry tincture is often made with whiskey or bourbon to honor the traditions and time-honored medicinal ways of working with colds. Think of a hot toddy "whiskey in hot tea." My lemon balm tincture uses a milder alcohol such as gin because it does not require a high level of alcohol to process it. This tincture also complements the flavor of the plant giving it a Fruity Pebbles cereal flavor.

This medicine-making tradition depended on the accessibility of the materials and that, in turn, depended on money, location, and the practitioner's training.

Making tinctures can get very technical, depending on your level of expertise. Folk traditions are a simplified process of this way of making medicine. I have loved to see how these traditions have expanded (and gotten more detailed) in order to create medicines for holistic healing.

Tincture Process

Supplies to make a tincture according to the folk method:

clean and sterile mason jars; depending on the amount of tincture you are making, use a half-pint, pint, or quart jar

scissors or knife for chopping the plant material

alcohol, vegetable glycerin, or apple cider vinegar

plant material—roots, combination of the aerial parts (parts that grow above ground—stem, fruit, leaf, bark, flower—and the seeded part)

basket, pillowcase, or another container to take the plants home in

Note: If you are harvesting or foraging your own plants, make sure you know the plant and how to properly identify it. An important message about working with the plants: bring an offering such as tobacco, a prayer, tiny crystals, or something that resonates with you to thank mother earth and the plant for their medicine. Always take a moment to talk with the plant before harvesting it, even if what you say is only a simple "thank you for your medicine." I feel that when we communicate about what we are going to do with a plant before we take it, this adds to the vibration of the medicine. No one—even a plant—likes to be forced into doing something. Giving thanks and saying prayers for the earth helps raise the plants' vibrations and honors the process it took to grow, from seed to harvest. This helps acknowledge the plant and the healing it will provide and is an important aspect of the process of making medicines.

If you are ordering your herbs online, make sure you learn as much about the supplier as possible. Contact them and ask questions. I feel that herbs from online sources deserve the same reverence as herbs you harvest on your own. Most suppliers are not aware that large-scale commercial harvesting uses unethical methods such as slave labor with mistreatment of workers, low to no pay for their work, and unsanitary working environments. The horror stories I have heard would shock most people, like used baby diapers being found in large bundles of plants as they arrive in the US. That is why it is important, when possible, to know the source of your herbs and seek out local herb farmers. I believe in being fully present when making herbal medicine by honoring the process and taking time to "cleanse" any negativity from myself and my space, as well as blessing the hands that planted and harvested the herbs. Using incense to bless the area, prayer, and song are very important. Doing this will help create a more positive vibrational medicine with a deeper healing effect that is full of love.

WHEN TO HARVEST

* Choose a dry day after the dew has disappeared.
* Choose plants that are at least 6 feet from the road.
* Find clean plants. Do not wash the leaves or flowers because water or dampness could create mold.
* Never harvest all the plants in one location; leave some in place so they can keep growing and produce more plant babies.
* Harvest roots in the fall when the top or aerial part of the plant has died off. A fall root harvest is one of my favorites. The cold earth and digging them up helps remind us that even in our darkest times, magic and medicine are happening. We should be gentler with ourselves in those phases of our life when we think "nothing is happening." Make sure that you wash off soil and mud, and then pat them dry.
* Harvest bark in the fall or early spring.
* Harvest flowers when they are about to open, or right after.
* Harvest leaves at their peak, when they are most viable.

MAKING THE TINCTURE

1. Fill a jar ½ to ¾ of the way up with your choice of herb, like dandelion root, nettles, or passionflower.

2. Fill the jar the rest of the way up with your alcohol of choice (typically vodka) or glycerin until it is an inch above the plant material.

3. Leave a headspace, or space between the liquid and the top (typically from where the grooves of the mason jar start to form).

4. Label the jar with the date, type of herb, and type of solvent used.

5. Shake the jar periodically (daily or weekly); saying a prayer adds your juju into the medicine.

6. Allow it to sit somewhere out of direct sun; I let mine sit in a dark place, like a cabinet, that has a constant, cool temperature (not somewhere with temperatures that vary from too hot to too cold). I then wait two to six weeks. Afterward, I store the tincture in a cool, dark place.

 ✤ When using fresh herbs, fill the jar to the top with the herbs or plant material, and leave just a little space so you can top off the mixture with alcohol.

 ✤ When using dried plant material, fill the jar ⅔ of the way to allow expansion of the plant material when it rehydrates.

 ✤ Check your medicine often in the first week and add more solvent if needed.

Advanced Tincture Approach

A typical tincture of dried herbs is used with a 1:5 or (up to) 1:10 ratio (herb to glycerin or 80- to 100-proof vodka).

A tincture using fresh herbs is used with a 1:2 or up to 1:5 ratio of herb to liquid, and 100-proof vodka is suggested. Doing this is suggested because fresh herbs will release more moisture, causing a risk of your tincture becoming rancid (and a higher proportion of liquor will forestall this).

TINCTURE MEASUREMENT EXAMPLES:

- ❀ 1 ounce of dried herb to 5 ounces of liquid (1:5)
- ❀ 3 ounces of dried herb to 15 ounces of liquid (3:15)
- ❀ 3 ounces of fresh herb to 6 ounces of liquid (3:6)

Formula Inspirations

It is wise to make single tinctures and then create formulas by blending them together.

Antiviral: elderberry, plantain leaf, echinacea root and flower, nettles (I love to use bourbon for this recipe.)

Calm your nerves: milky oats, tulsi (holy basil), and passionflower

Women's balance support blend for menopausal issues : Vitex, black cohosh, and motherwort

How to Make Botanical-Infused Oils and Healing Salve Recipes

For over twenty-five years, I have been obsessed with creating infused botanical oils. In the spa industry, I was in training and development, working with many spas and companies to create unique experiences that indulge all the senses.

As a child, I learned from fashion magazines about different oils to slather myself with; then as an adult, I blended essential oils into shea butter and various oil bases for everyone. When I think back, rose oil was the first oil I infused with botanicals. Then, as I learned about the plant world, my knowledge expanded even further.

I found I could layer different textures of oils with plants, including plantain leaf (the weed, not the fruit) for soothing skin; violet leaf for breast massaging and my famous vaginal lube; comfrey leaf for just about everything from sore muscles to skin issues; calendula for babies' skin products and adding a nourishing glow to adult skin. The inspirations, healing properties, and recipes are endless, so endless that aside from some bath products, I have almost stopped using essential oils altogether. After ending up with chemical burns using essential oil skincare products purchased from "natural product" lines, I find fewer reactions ensue from herbal-infused skin care.

When you love the plants and the earth, you start to think about overharvesting and sustainability. It takes 22 pounds of rose petals to produce one 5-milliliter bottle of rose essential oil. DO YOU KNOW HOW MUCH MEDICINE I COULD MAKE FROM 22 POUNDS OF ROSES? I could make teas, tinctures, cordials, spiritual baths, gallons of infused oils, and so much more—much more than I could get from that five-milliliter bottle of essential oil!

I often think of the "old timey" folkways of my ancestors, such as using animal fat to infuse plants to treat ailments. Some healers still practice those techniques today. Recently I saw an ad for someone selling plant medicine infused with bear fat. Emma Dupree spoke of using turtle fat for arthritis. I imagine my ancestors slow-cooking over a fire or wood stove until they were sure that all the herbs' medicine was infused in the fat.

Choosing the Right Oil for Your Infusion

Choosing the right oil for what you want to use it for is important. I love using only food-grade oils. Heavy olive oil in a face serum could clog the pores of many skin types. However, that same oil could be a good base for an infusion used in making salves because that oil would hold the plant medicine topically: oils with more fat content stay on the skin surface longer than oils with less fat content, thus creating a topical pain reliever. Coconut oil strengthens connective tissues, and this oil, along with and grape-seed oil, acts as skin food. I love to layer oils of different textures; each formula has a unique feel and benefit when applied to skin. Here are a few of my favorite ones to use for both their medical and magical properties for skin care as well as for cooking. I love to find all the easy ways to add plant medicine to every part of my life I can. Let's get started!

Avocado oil—this super-rich oil is a beautiful addition to dryer skin. I love its rich texture when paired with a lighter oil like grape seed. It contains goodness like beta carotene, protein, and fatty acids, along with vitamins A, D, and E to help moisturize and protect your skin from ultraviolet rays' damage; it also increases collagen metabolism.

Baobab oil—this comes from a tree nicknamed "the tree of life" because most will live for over five hundred years. The powder of the tree's fruit is used in food, but the oil is used mostly in skin and body care products because it has moisturizing properties and is packed with vitamins B and C, and omega 3. It also has anti-inflammatory benefits, making it a choice for those sensitive to other oils. It is also great to use for hair, skin, and nails.

Castor oil—this oil comes from seeds of the *Ricinus communis* plant, which is native to tropical areas of Africa and Asia. Castor oil is thought to have anti-inflammatory, antimicrobial moisturizing properties, and is good for sprains and swollen joints. It is also used in "packs" or as a poultice (this is a topical remedy that uses a small cloth soaked in the oil and covered with another cloth and a hot water bottle to help it penetrate into the skin tissue even deeper). I use this poultice often on my hands for the repetitive strain injury that comes from years of working as an aesthetician in a spa.

Castor oil was used for stomach issues and often given orally by the elders to so many of us with Southern roots. Modern research shows that castor oil is broken down into ricinoleic acid in the small intestine.[28] This speeds up the process of digestion. Oh, the stories from elders about lining up at home so their grandmothers could dose them with this can be heard throughout the South. The faces they make when recounting those times of their childhood are priceless.

Coconut oil—this oil is high in vitamins E and K, and it has antifungal and antibacterial properties. Remember to look for cold-pressed, unrefined coconut oil for your face or skin care.

Grape-seed oil—this is lighter than jojoba oil or coconut oil, and thus better at controlling facial oils. It also has a lot of vitamin E, about twice as much as olive oil has! This means it provides antioxidants for your skin, which could help with damage from free radicals. As an aesthetician, I loved this oil for problematic skin because of its ability to help oily and acne-prone skin stay hydrated, balancing oil production and not causing irritation. This oil is high in linoleic acid, which is thought to reduce clogged pores.

Olive oil—this oil is most loved as the base oil infusion used in salves and topical medicinal oils; its higher fat content lets the plant medicine stay on the surface of the skin instead of being absorbed more quickly as oils with less fat content do. Olive oil contains vitamins A, D, E, and K.

Rosehip seed oil—this oil is extracted from the seeds of a South American rosebush; rosehip seed oil is like Mother Nature's Retin-A, without the irritating side effects. It contains omega-6 essential fatty acids and vitamins A and C, which increase cell turnover. If you use it for a few weeks, you may notice a lightning effect in any dark spots, smoothing of scars, or balancing of any other skin discoloration.

This retinol-like effect and the resulting increase in collagen and elastin production means that aging skin will benefit from this oil too. The oil's high concentrations of linoleic acid may also help with uneven pigmentation, scars, fine lines, and acne-prone skin.

---

28 Aaron Kandola, "Benefits of Castor Oil for the Face and Skin," *Medical News Today* (June 28, 2018), https://www.medicalnewstoday.com/articles/319844.

Shea butter—this is a natural vegetable fat that comes from shea tree nuts, and most of it is used in food. It has potent anti-inflammatory and antioxidant properties, which makes it amazing for skin. According to the Center for the Promotion of Imports Ministry of Foreign Affairs,[29] two types exist: Western African shea butter and East African shea butter.

It is in hair treatments for damaged and dry hair, in anti-aging and anti-wrinkle creams, and in body creams; this oil is also used for sunburn care, in diaper rash creams, and in bases for pain salves.

WESTERN AFRICAN SHEA BUTTER	EAST AFRICAN SHEA BUTTER
❁ Higher concentration of vitamin ❁ Higher melting point ❁ Lower concentration of oleic acid ❁ Harder in consistency ❁ Higher concentration of sterol	❁ More yellow in color ❁ Lower melting point ❁ Higher concentration of leic acid ❁ Soft and creamy texture

Sunflower seed oil—high in vitamin E and lightweight, this oil is one of my new favorites. I love to look at sunflowers, so I imagine adding that bright sunny when I use this oil in my formulations.

Choosing the Right Plants

Here are some of my favorite herbs, weeds, leaves, flowers, and tree bark to use in plant medicine:

---

29 "The European Market Potential for Shea Butter," CBI Ministry of Foreign Affairs, last updated February 10, 2021, https://www.cbi.eu/market-information/natural-ingredients -cosmetics/shea-butter/market-potential. See Hana Ames, "What Are the Benefits of Shea Butter?" *Medical News Today*, April 21, 2021, https://www.medicalnewstoday.com/articles /shea-butter-benefits#types.

For Skin

arnica (for pain)

calendula (is anti-inflammatory; for keeping skin healthy and moisturized; is great to use in children's skincare)

comfrey (for muscle sprains, healthy skin, and healing wounds)

hemp (for balancing oil production and calming; helps reduce fine lines. CBD oil is often used in topical pain products as well.)

peach tree leaves (soothes and calms skin; is also said to have antioxidant properties)

plantain leaf (for skin soothing)

rose (for skin hydration, calming, and increasing circulation in the skin)

St. John's wort flowers (has wound-healing properties and helps calm acne, eczema, and dry skin)

violet leaf and flower (for lymphatic flow; is great for breast massage products)

willow bark (for pain)

For Food

dandelion root

holy basil

nettles

vitex

Solar-Infused Oils

Process these herb-infused oils by using the heat from sunlight to infuse the properties of the herbs into the oil. You will need the following supplies:

herb of choice (either fresh—wilted—or dried)

wide-mouth jars of various sizes—2 ounces to 32 ounces, with tight-fitting caps (sterile)

oil of choice

knife

scissors

label

dish or saucer for catching oil drops while the oil sets

cloth to cover and protect the oil from light

cheesecloth or jelly bag, colander

Techniques for Preparing Infused Oils

Mold is a common problem when introducing water-rich, juicy plant material to an oil base. I learned this by infusing fresh flowers into oils; I lost an entire jar of honeysuckle oil the first time I tried it. Practice with other plant-infused oils, and then try infusing the oil with fresh flowers.

You want to pick the leaves or flowers after the dew has dried but before the sun has heated the plant because the heat from the sun will release the vital aromatic oils. I learned about this while I was in Thailand.

1. Remove any bruised or discolored material and set the plant material out for 24 hours (this is called dry wilting).

2. Tear, cut, or chop the herbs in small pieces, and choose the size of jar appropriate for the amount of herb.

3. Fill the jar 1 inch from the top with fresh plant material. If using dried herbs, fill the jar only ⅓ full.

4. Fill the jar with the oil. Make sure you fill the jar to the very top.

5. There must be enough oil to completely cover the herbs. This will ensure no mold or bacterial growth will grow on the top of the setting herbs.

6. Cover tightly with the mason jar lid.

7. Place the jar in a warm (not hot), sunny location. Let the jar sit sheltered from direct sun or covered with cloth for 2 weeks. (Check occasionally for any drop in oil level; add more oil if needed.)

8. Place a dish towel under the infusing oils, as they sometimes leak during the process.

9. After 2 weeks, strain out the herbs (compost strained herbs) using a cheesecloth or jelly bag. Do not squeeze herbs that have been used when fresh because they contain small amounts of water and this will cause the oils to get moldy.

10. If you want to add fragrance to your oils, do so now before storing them.

11. Label and store the oil in either amber or dark-colored glass containers in a dark and dry place for 6 months to 3 years. Some herbal oils last longer than others; routinely check on them to smell if they have gone rancid.

Double Boiler Method—this is an infusion method consisting of two saucepans fitting together so that the contents of the upper pan can be heated by boiling water in the lower pan. This is the best method to use when you need oils in a hurry.

1. Prepare and place the herb or herbs in a double boiler.

2. Cover the herbs with oil, making sure at least 1 to 2 inches of extra oil top the herbs.

3. Cover and simmer on low for 1 to 4 hours.

4. Strain and bottle.

5. Add essential oils after straining (optional).

6. Label and store as above.

Water Bath Method—This is an infusion method whereby a large mason jar is placed into a Crock-Pot full of water on its lowest setting (warm) to infuse for 2 to 3 days. DO NOT place a lid on the jar for safety reasons; it will cause heat, pressure, and moisture buildup. Fill the water in the Crock-Pot up to the level of oil and add water as needed so your oil infusion will be heated evenly. Check on it and stir often. Use caution if you choose to leave it on overnight for fire safety reasons.

My Favorite Recipes: using equal parts of each herb and filling up the jar with the chosen oil or combinations of oils.

Note: For oil to relieve pain, I prefer olive because it sits on the skin.

Note: For topical skin serum, I prefer a combination of oils, usually three different ones tailored to the skin, each used to produce better texture, to nourish the skin, and to help treat specific skin issues.

For pain relief—comfrey, St. John's wort, willow bark, hemp

For soothing skin—comfrey, plantain, calendula, rose

SALVE MAKING MADE EASY

A salve is a topical ointment used to soothe the skin, draw out infection, or relieve pain. Different herbs produce different results. Black ointment (also called drawing salve) has been traditionally used to treat minor skin problems, such as sebaceous cysts, boils, in-grown toenails, and splinters. Choose one herbal-infused oil or a combination of a few to treat specific issues, such as pain, or skin problems, such as irritation. Be careful with this one and use formulas only from a reputable source. It can be quite powerful and irritate the skin.

1 ounce beeswax (use shea butter for a vegan salve)

4 ounces herbal-infused oil(s) of your choice

10 to 20 drops essential oil of choice (optional)

1. Wrap the beeswax bar in an old towel. Place it on a sturdy surface like a cutting board and use a hammer to break up the bar into smaller chunks. I prefer the pellets because they are ready to be measured and melt more quickly.

2. Place the beeswax in a double boiler (I sometimes just use a larger pot less than half full of water and place a Pyrex bowl over that to create a double boiler) and slowly warm the beeswax over low heat until it melts. Do not rush the process.

3. Add in your premade herbal-infused oils and stir the mixture over low heat until it is well blended.

4. Remove from the heat.

5. Add the essential oil(s), if using, for extra aroma.

6. Quickly pour the warm mixture into prepared tins, or glass or plastic jars. You can also create fabulous lip balms by purchasing tubes or even smaller containers and putting the mixture in these containers.

7. Let the mixture cool completely; it will become solid.

8. Store in a cool location for 1 to 3 years.

Tea Time! Folk Remedies and How to Create Tea Blends for Wellness

Herbal teas have been one of the most common ways to benefit from plant medicine. An herbal tea is a blend of herbs, flowers, spices, roots, bark, and/or dried fruit. If you harvest your own plants and have limited resources, you pretty much can help heal yourself with the teas; they are great if you are on a budget because all you do is add water and love. The elders would use teas as treatment for many illnesses. Teas of life everlasting are important to the Gullah Geechee people; the elders believe when you take this you will not get sick. Yellow root was a go-to remedy for many people in the South as soon as they felt any illness coming on—you see Emma Dupree making this tea in her documentary "Little Medicine Thing." Sassafras tea was a main ingredient in a Southern house apothecary for the cold season.

Some time ago, I was living in New Orleans and running around the swamps studying plants used by the Maroons, who were descendants of African Americans who often mixed with the indigenous people to form settlements to escape from being enslaved. It was fascinating to see how they would have lived using the resources from the area to survive and hide. There I learned from the elders about using Spanish moss tea for fevers, chills, birth pangs, and menopausal issues. The Gullah Geechee and the indigenous peoples also widely used this remedy. Spanish moss also helped with skin issues, body pains, and arthritis. Many people would slowly steep Spanish moss tea on their wood stoves, over a fire, or in more modern times, on a stovetop until they were rich in color— that was the time to "pull the medicine out" of the tea.

A cup of tea is amazing in so many ways. It can warm your bones on a cold night, bring you a little respite from a hard day, and be a quick fix for what ails you. Some cultures, such as Haitian, have teas in which you can use only one leaf in a cup because it is so strong—enough to "pull the fever out."

I love using herbal infusions to reap the full benefits of plant medicine. Herbal teas use less plant matter and are steeped for a shorter period of time—three to fifteen minutes, while herbal infusions use a larger quantity of herbs and are steeped longer. I like to prepare my herbal infusions the night before, allowing them to steep in a mason jar anywhere from four to eight hours to make a powerful medicine. I find myself feeling my best when I consume them regularly, drinking a quart jar a day, rotating my recipes to specific issues I am dealing with. Or I have my favorite blend that is my go-to most of the time. I will share the recipe with you on "My Favorite Herbal Tea Blends" on page 102.

I also love a good sun tea when it is summertime and you have the perfect spot to let the heat of the sun work its magic. Nothing to me says "Southern" like a pitcher of solar-infused sweet tea poured over a glass of ice on a hot summer day!

I have so many fond memories of sun tea as a child. I would often check on it many times during the process to watch the color get richer and richer until dinnertime, when we could drink it. My mother had a special tea container, with a spout on it, just for sun tea.

When I think about the energy that the sun gives to plant medicine, it truly warms my soul.

HERB/WATER RATIO (for medicinal-strength teas):

⚜ 1 to 2 tablespoons dry plants or herbs: 1 cup water

⚜ 3 to 4 tablespoons fresh plants or herbs: 1 cup water

For larger quantities:

⚜ 1 ounce or 1 cup dried herbs or plant material: 1 quart water

⚜ 2 ounces or 2 cups fresh herbs or plant material: 1 quart water

FOR CHRONIC PROBLEMS: Suggested use is 3 to 4 cups a day, 5 days a week. This protocol can be extended for a few weeks if needed. Then, give the body a break while using other teas for other issues you may have. I use the balancing infusion almost daily, then switch to the Immunitea (see below) if a cold starts coming on.

ACUTE PROBLEMS: Suggested use is ¼ to ½ cup every 30 minutes till symptoms subside.

MY FAVORITE HERBAL TEA BLENDS

These blends can also be used as inspirations for tincture formulas.

Balancing infusion: equal parts nettles, holy basil, and milky oats, and ½ part rose petals

Immunitea: equal parts of elderberry, nettles, Reishi mushroom, and ginger

Just chill (adult sleepy time): equal parts skullcap, passionflower, and peppermint

Love yourself: equal parts hawthorn, linden, and rose

Relax for children: equal parts lemon balm and chamomile (omit if you have a ragweed allergy)

Pine needle tea (for cold and flu season to help support immune system): use white pine needles, rinsed and chopped (you can also use pine combs that still have some resin in them; do not use the brown ones)

Antioxidant boost tea: equal parts peach and blueberry leaves (also great infused in an oil for skin)

Smoke Blends

Some herb blends used in ceremonies and to treat ailments are smoked in a pipe or rolled into a cigarette. These smoke blends help people with respiratory issues, including quitting smoking tobacco by supporting the lungs during the process. Herbs used include mullein and life everlasting (a.k.a. rabbit tobacco).

One of my favorite blends is mullein, peppermint, rose, and life everlasting. Remove the stems and grind up the mixture. As you sip a cup of tea, enjoy this blend in meditation or in a sacred circle of friends on the porch or by the fire.

CHAPTER 6

IN THE HEALING KITCHENS OF OUR GRANDMOTHERS

I teach a lot about ancestor connection, food, and plant medicine in herbal schools, to my own students and at conferences. It is through the plants that I have learned about the ancestors of my culture and have felt connected. I love to inspire students to interview their families and find out more about them through their connection to food traditions. Food and sharing stories about food with families and communities connects us in ways that can heal us.

I had a client who came to me after a lecture to ask about connecting to her ancestors. Her mom had a mental illness and traumatic childhood, so it was uncomfortable for her mom to talk about it. She would just shut down. I suggested asking her mother about her favorite meal that her own mother had cooked for her. I call them my ancestors' meals. That is the meal that instantly takes you back to childhood. We may all have some trauma, but most of us can remember at least one good meal with our family. My client wrote to me a week later and said she had been on the phone with her mother for two hours, talking about food memories. You could feel her spirit glow through her words.

I had another client whose mother had a stroke, and the pressure of switching caregiving roles was bringing up emotions. Her mother felt like she had no purpose. I suggested that they begin a different way of spending time by sharing stories. My client knew very little about her own grandparents. I suggested easing into talking about them by asking her mother to talk about the food she remembered her mother making for her. It worked. Thanks to these conversations, my client learned many things. She discovered her mother's joy telling those stories. My client also realized that she herself was a legacy herbalist, one who loved to forge for herbs and food—a beloved practice of their ancestors.

Reflection: What memories do you have about a meal in your childhood? Ask your parents or grandparents. Write their answers down.

As I get older, I realize the importance of heirloom recipes and writing them down. Losing my grandmother in my twenties was extremely difficult, and there is not a single picture of me as a child where I was not standing in my grandmother's kitchen. I would be on that yellow linoleum floor right next to her, sampling food and seeing all the delicious ways that she showed love to all of us through her food. My time in the kitchen is my time to express ancestor love with traditions used for generations. Growing up in my grandmother's kitchen and being always by her side, I learned early on about the ways we can show our love through cooking.

It took what seems most of the rest of my life to come to terms with grief and turn cooking into a way to remember my grandmother, and not the trauma of losing her. When I am practicing these ways, I communicate with her by remembering how her hands would go through the same processes of each thing I create. It is my sacred space with my ancestors. I love to honor the old ways and then put a twist of plant medicine in my food, not only to help heal my body but also to weave in the magic of the plants. Some say we cook and conjure with every dish.

Most of us who grew up in the South remember how we would come together on the farm as a community to harvest, process, and preserve the fruits of our summer labor on the land. It was hard work and at times I did not understand how important this rite of passage was. It was the time when the women got together on the front porch to talk, and if you were quiet, you got to hear the pearls of knowledge passed back and forth, to hear the family gossip, the "grown folks business."

What had been a Southern child's nightmare of full harvest has become my most fond memory. It is my life's work to inspire others to return to these ways, bringing families and communities together. I want to inspire people to share the stories of their people who so beautifully loved each of us through the work in the kitchen; I want to help people remember the times they may have forgotten.

Most of us have spent our childhoods in kitchens standing next to our grandmothers, clutching their apron strings. We should bring back these old ways to honor these women, their legacy of love; our food can heal us and our families. So many people have wandered so far away from what real food is and where it comes from, and it is exciting to see people making their way back home.

Many indigenous cultures understood the importance of food as the key to health and wellness. But it was more than just the food alone. They had reverence for the entire process, from honoring the land in which food is grown, to planting the seed, to caring for the crop and the animals, to singing the sweet songs of harvest.

Knowing about and honoring the process is especially important if you are not connected to the farm that you get your food from. This lack creates a disconnect between food and the act of consuming. Also, some farms still use "slave labor" practices and have harsh working environments, and that negative energy goes into the food. With better kitchen practices and more attention paid to where we purchase our food, things could start to change: food grown under the right circumstances is like an energetic cleanse of your produce, meat, and herbs, better activating their nutritional and medicinal potential. Coming back to the old ways by using food from small local farms and honoring folk traditions, and combining these actions with plant medicine, magic, love, and the healing arts, we can create holistic alchemy in all our food!

These pages are dedicated to our mothers' mothers' mothers, those who worked and still work the land, those who loved us through their food, the ways of our ancestors, and the healing magic in us all. Join me on this journey as we take a closer look at how we can connect more deeply to the process of preparing our food as sacred medicine—and enjoying some of my favorite heirloom recipes that have a modern twist.

Creating the Sacred Space

Many cultures understand that to create the best medicines for healing, you must create the best space energetically to prepare them.

This helps us understand that preparing a meal can be more than assembling ingredients—it is a way to honor and connect with ancestors, and music has always been there for this journey. From the ancient harvest songs of the Motherland, to the chants to honor all our devotion to our spirituality and the divine forces, to the old Negro spirituals sung at church, to the cadences in the fields that held secret messages for escaping slavery, music has always been there for the journey.

What songs remind you of your ancestors? Feel free to discover your own rhythm through a playlist that brings joy to your heart; write a few in your journal space or recipe book and share your playlist with family.

I also enjoy setting up sacred space by lighting candles, saying prayers that involve saying ancestors' names, cooking meals they would have prepared, and sometimes, just having pictures of them in my kitchen and medicine-making spaces.

When I am thinking about preparing old family recipes, I love to listen to old-school music. One song that is on my playlist that inspires me is Sam Cooke's "Bring It on Home to Me." What is on your playlist to remind you of memories of cooking with your family?

Kitchen Medicine to Fight the Funk

Long before the days of over-the-counter medicines, kitchen and herbal remedies were all people had, and they depended on them for the health and wellness of the family. They were used as preventive medicines to ward off illnesses and, when needed, to fight colds and other common ailments. These recipes are steeped in the folk medicine traditions and differ from household to household, depending on what was available at the time. I have added my own twist to them and as you get comfortable with creating them, you will explore and add your own as well.

GRANNY'S ONION COUGH SYRUP

Depending on the amount you want to make, this recipe is easy to alter. You can use more onions or fewer if you want a small batch for yourself. This is one of the recipes that Mary Hayden used during the 1918 Flu Pandemic as a primary medicine; she used easily available resources. She cut up onions, added sugar, and roasted them in an oven.

My granny taught me to decoct or simmer the onions slowly and on low heat. Then, as I always do, I took her recipe and combined it with other plant allies to make one beautiful medicine rooted in the love of our grandmothers' hands and hearts. I use this ancestor concoction every time I start to feel the funk of sickness. Onions have antiviral properties. In the South they were used for many illnesses and to help fight fever. When our grandmothers learned a child was sick with fever, they would slice onions, take the child's socks off, place those onions slices on the child's feet, and put their socks back on while rocking them and humming those songs to them the way only they could do it. Our grandmothers would pet the child's head and talk the fever out.

Grandmothers also used onions as a poultice on the chest for respiratory issues. Here's a recipe for granny's onion cough syrup. I prefer Vidalia onions because that is what I grew up on, but you can use whatever you have on hand. Instead of raw sugar, you can also add honey, maple syrup, agave, or stevia.

2 to 3 onions, sliced

¼ to ½ cup raw sugar

1 cinnamon stick (optional)

1 tablespoon sassafras (optional)

1 tablespoon wild cherry bark (optional)

1 tablespoon mullein (optional)

1 inch fresh ginger, grated or chopped (optional)

1. Put everything in a medium pot.

2. Add enough water to cover the ingredients.

3. Put on a lid and bring the mixture to a light boil.

4. Reduce the temperature and simmer on low heat for 30 to 45 minutes.

5. Strain the mixture into a mason jar and store in the refrigerator for up to 5 days.

6. Take 1 to 2 tablespoons 3 to 4 times daily with a prayer for healing.

ELDERBERRY SYRUP

This powerful and popular folk remedy has been used in households for quite some time to fight off colds and flu germs. Elderberries are amazing for boosting the immune system. Some families line up and take small daily doses before leaving the house each day. You can customize the syrup to suit your family's taste. I sometimes add a few tablespoons of lemon balm for families with children. It also has antiviral properties and is amazing for children who are a little more active and nervous. I feel children need a little plant medicine to help with stress during these modern times. Lemon balm alone is also a plant medicine I love in tea or glycerin (a tincture made with vegetable glycerin instead of alcohol) for children who are grieving. Dried ginger has a stronger flavor than fresh ginger, so adjust the amounts accordingly. Add more honey to increase the shelf life, and do not use honey for children under the age of one.

3 cups water

1½ cups dried or 2 cups fresh elderberries

½- to 1-inch fresh ginger, grated or roughly chopped (optional)

2 tablespoons dried nettles (optional)

2 tablespoons dried lemon balm

1 cinnamon stick

2-inch Reishi mushroom slice (optional)

1 cup raw local honey (or your favorite sweetener)

1. Place the water, elderberries, ginger (if using), nettles (if using), lemon balm, cinnamon stick, and Reishi mushroom slice in a saucepan over medium heat.

2. Bring the mixture to a slight boil, reduce the heat to low, and simmer for 30 minutes.

3. Turn the heat off and allow the mixture to sit for an hour.

4. Use a potato masher to mash the berries to release the juice; strain the mixture through a fine sieve or use a doubled cheesecloth, retaining juice and discarding the pulp.

5. Let the juice cool slightly, add the honey, and stir well.

6. Store the syrup in your refrigerator for up to 6 months; make sure the lid is on tight and that you label the container with the date you made it and what it is.

Note: I take 1 to 2 teaspoons daily for illness prevention.

FIRE CIDER

According to old folk remedies, this is said to be an anti-viral as well as a great decongestant, among other things.

Fire cider also helps supports the immune system and can aid with digestion. Substitute the jalapeno pepper with Scotch, bonnet, or habanero if you love more heat. You can make small to large batches of this recipe, depending on your needs, by adjusting the amounts of the ingredients. I make a gallon at a time to last me all winter! Have fun with it! You can also use fresh herbs like rosemary and thyme.

½ cup grated fresh horseradish

1 to 2 medium onions, sliced

1 to 2 cloves garlic, crushed or chopped

¼ teaspoon (or more) cayenne pepper

1 jalapeno pepper

1 to 2 lemons, limes, or oranges, juiced; reserve the peel

½ cup grated or chopped fresh ginger

2 to 3 tablespoons dried hibiscus flowers (optional)

1 tablespoon ground turmeric, 1 inch fresh turmeric, chopped, or 2 dried turmeric roots

1 bottle organic raw, unfiltered apple cider vinegar

¼ cup honey (or more to taste)

1. Place all the ingredients, except the vinegar and the honey, in a quart jar.

2. Pour in the apple cider vinegar, covering all the ingredients.

3. Cover the jar with a plastic lid, or put parchment paper over the top of the jar, and screw on the metal lid (the paper helps prevent the lid from rusting).

4. Shake well.

5. Store in a dark, cool, and dry space for a month, shaking the jar at least three times a week.

6. When it is ready, strain the ingredients using a doubled cheesecloth or fine strainer, pressing out all the liquid. Add the honey (to taste) and mix well (you can also substitute your favorite sweetener).

7. Take one shot daily.

Note: I prefer to cook with it. It is amazing over greens and many other things! I also make my salad dressings with it.

EASY BONE BROTH

This may be anti-aging because bone broth is associated with collagen, a protein found in skin, cartilage, and bone; it is good for digestion and gut health and helps support immune system function. Ask your butcher to cut the best beef bones for soup into smaller pieces or in half. When using chicken bones, I like to use the bones from a rotisserie chicken. I prefer the no-salt version of Tony Chachere's seasoning, my go-to spice after living in New Orleans. Reduce the garlic, if desired, smashing the cloves and using the skins.

organic beef soup bones

4 carrots, chopped

3 celery stalks, chopped

2 medium onions, skins on

2 bay leaves

1 head garlic

handful dried nettles

2 sprigs fresh rosemary

5 sprigs fresh thyme

4-inch slice dried Reishi mushroom

½ teaspoon black or white pepper, or both

½ to 1 teaspoon Tony Chachere's No Salt Seasoning Blend seasoning or your favorite spice blend

2 to 3 tablespoons olive oil

1 to 2 (32-ounce) containers stock or broth (optional)

1 tablespoon apple cider vinegar

1. Preheat the oven to 450°F.

2. On a baking sheet, arrange the beef bones, cut vegetables, garlic, and herbs. Season with the pepper and the seasoning blend; drizzle with a little olive oil; and mix (if you are using leftover rotisserie chicken bones, you do not have to roast those bones; just add them to the liquid).

3. Roast this mixture for 30 minutes; then gently flip the mixture and roast for 15 to 20 more minutes.

4. Remove the mixture from the pan and add to a stockpot or pots if you need to make a larger batch. I like to use my Instant Pot; it is quicker and less trouble (see the instructions for making bone broth in the Instant Pot or slow cooker on page 114). If you are using chicken bones, add the bones now.

5. Cover the mixture with water; I like to add extra flavor, so I add 1 to 2 32-ounce containers of stock and fill the pot the rest of the way with water until the bones are fully submerged.

6. Add 1 tablespoon of apple cider vinegar to help break the bones down.

Instructions for the Instant Pot

1. Fill the container to 1 inch below "Max" line.

2. Make sure your sealing ring is in place on the lid. Lock the lid onto the Instant Pot and set the steam release knob to the "sealing" position.

3. Press the "manual" button and set your Instant Pot for high pressure for 120 minutes. (I find it easier to decrease the time because the timer resets at 120 after you decrease to zero.) It will take about 15 to 30 minutes for the Instant Pot to come to full pressure, then the display will show a countdown timer.

4. Once the two hours are up, allow the pressure to release naturally. It will take about 15 to 30 minutes.

5. Strain the broth through a doubled cheesecloth or a strainer and allow to cool. The broth will usually have a layer of fat on the top and will gelatinize when thoroughly cooled. Remove the fat with a spoon and discard (some people love to cook with the fat).

Instructions for Stovetop

1. Add the broth ingredients to a stockpot and simmer over medium-high heat, then reduce the heat to as low as your stove will go. You want the broth to be just barely bubbling. Cover with the lid slightly ajar and cook for 24 hours for poultry bones and 48 hours for red-meat bones. You can place the whole pot (covered) in the fridge overnight and resume cooking the broth in the morning.

2. Strain the broth when it has finished cooking.

3. Store the broth in mason jars for up to 5 days in your refrigerator. Or divide it into small portions (for easy access) and freeze for up to 6 months.

Instructions for the Slow Cooker

1. Cover the pot with the lid slightly ajar, and cook on low for 24 hours for poultry bones and on low for 48 hours for red meat bones. Due to possible fire hazard, use caution if you leave your Crock-Pot or slow cooker on overnight.

VEGAN MEDICINAL MUSHROOM BROTH

To make this broth, I usually use just Reishi mushrooms but when I add all three, I feel like it is a super blend. But Reishi will always be my first mushroom love. You can make Lucretia's Kickin' Creole Seasoning (see page 124) instead of using Tony Chachere's seasoning; add more spices for more flavor.

3 carrots, chopped

3 celery stalks, chopped

1 large onion, skins on

up to 1 head of garlic, smashed, with skins on

olive oil

2 bay leaves

1 to 2 (32-ounce) containers vegetable broth or stock (enough to cover all the ingredients)

2 slices dried Reishi mushrooms or a combo of my favorite powerful fungi: Reishi (*Ganoderma lucidum/ tsugae*), chaga (*Inotus obliquus*), and turkey tail (*Trametes versicolor*)

handful dried nettles

2 sprigs fresh rosemary

4 sprigs fresh thyme

½ teaspoon black or white pepper (I use both)

½ inch fresh turmeric root or ½ teaspoon ground turmeric

½ to 1 teaspoon Tony Chachere's No Salt Seasoning Blend seasoning (optional)

pinch cayenne (optional)

1 to 2 (3-inch) sticks yellow root (optional)

1. Roast the cut vegetables and garlic, drizzled with olive oil, on a baking pan at 450°F for 30 minutes, turning the mixture halfway through the cooking time.

2. Put the vegetable mixture in a pot and add enough water or stock to cover all vegetables.

3. Add the medicinal mushrooms, herbs, yellow root, and seasonings.

4. Bring the mixture to a boil, cover with a lid, reduce the heat, and simmer for 3 hours.

5. Strain and store the broth in mason jars, or you can divide the broth into small portions and freeze it.

6. Once the broth cools, reheat it as needed.

7. You can also use an Instant Pot. Just set the timer for 1 hour on the "soup" setting and allow it to self vent.

TIP

Save all vegetable scraps from cooking in a freezer bag to add extra flavor to these bone and mushroom broth recipes.

Soul Food with a Little Vegan Twist

Michael Twitty, a food writer, author, and bearer of Black food traditions, said in the Netflix series *High on the Hog*: "We are the only people who named our cuisine after something invisible that you could feel, love and God; it is the connection between us and our dead and with those waiting to be born."[30] That quote hit me so deep! Our food is so deep and rich in our traditions that it started a "soul food" movement. Its food is so good and full of so much love that it goes straight to the soul, an unseen part of the body that could only be felt. I enjoyed the series so much I had to buy the book that inspired it.

30 "High on the Hog," episode 2.

In that book, *High on the Hog: A Culinary Journey from Africa to America*, Jessica B. Harris takes us on a culinary journey to Africa, into the markets and traditions of the Motherland, through the Middle Passage, and into the spaces of the enslaved chefs who helped begin the soul food movement. Just like the research of our story of herbal medicine, this research about soul food made me aware of the complexity of our journey with food, what it took to make those dishes we all know and love, like macaroni and cheese.

Harris writes about the foods that made it over from Africa, like okra, black-eyed peas (in Africa, they are used for luck and to ward off negative energies), and watermelon. These were the "gifts" Africans brought into the New World. She describes how food was the only piece of home that people brought with them.[31]

I grew up in the South, and soul food has been a part of my entire life. One of my most favorite meals is pinto beans, collard greens, and corn bread with lots of fire cider and hot sauce! It is so simple, but it takes me back! As an adult, I travel so much and I always love to find the food I grew on. Cooking traditions change but, at the same time, are honored. I chose to add a vegan twist—that is to say, an option—to the recipes in this chapter to introduce ways to change up from the heavy meat-based diets of the South. I spent a few years being plant based and found that it was a wonderful challenge to re-create old heirloom recipes of my youth and then add a dollop of herbal medicine.

31 Jessica B. Harris, *High on the Hog: A Culinary Journey from Africa to America* (New York: Bloomsbury, 2012).

Soul Food Recipes

VEGAN COLLARD GREENS WITH POTLICKER

You can also use 1 to 2 tablespoons of dried herbs like vitex, nettles—which you can use fresh—and dandelion root for extra plant medicine.

2 pounds washed and cut collard, mustard, or turnip greens, or a combination

2 onions, peeled and diced

6 cloves garlic, peeled and finely chopped

3 tablespoons olive oil

2 to 3 pinches red pepper flakes

4 to 5 pinches smoked paprika

2 to 3 pinches black and/or white pepper

1 to 2 pinches salt

2 teaspoons liquid smoke (optional)

3 to 4 cups vegetable stock or medicinal mushroom broth

hot sauce (optional)

dash of fire cider (optional)

1. Wash the collards thoroughly.

2. Roll up the leaves lengthwise and thinly slice them.

3. Sauté the onion and garlic in your stockpot with olive oil until you smell them, and they become translucent. Add the seasonings. (I keep adding seasoning throughout the cooking process until I get the flavor I want.)

4. Add in the sliced greens and cover with the stock or broth.

5. Bring the greens to a slight boil, cover, reduce the heat, and simmer for 1 to 3 hours, or until the greens reach the desired tenderness.

6. Add your favorite hot sauce and a dash of fire cider, if using.

7. Enjoy and make sure you get some of that juice called potlicker for extra medicinal love!

POKE SALAD A.K.A. SALLET

This recipe is a tradition in the South once springtime comes. One of the first plants to come up after the last frost of winter, poke is a strong lymphatic and used by families to help "clean" or move out of the body the rich foods of the winter. Use with caution and do not forget the first step to boil the leaves at least three times to remove excess toxins. To make this recipe vegan or vegetarian, omit the bacon. Vegans may also omit the fire cider if it contains honey.

poke greens (collect greens in the spring that are no higher than your knee)

3 to 4 slices bacon

1 small onion peeled, and sliced or diced

6 cloves garlic, minced

salt and pepper

smoked paprika

hot sauce

fire cider or vinegar (optional)

1. Pick poke when it is small enough to be tender. Parboil in enough water to cover the greens. Drain and rinse thoroughly; repeat this step one to two more times to reduce toxicity and until the greens are tender. Stain out as much water as you can. Doing this greatly reduces the amount of vitamin A in the leaves (this vitamin may be toxic at certain levels. Do not skip this step!)

2. Fry the bacon and save the grease to use later (use olive oil if vegan or vegetarian).

3. Sauté the onion and garlic.

4. Add the poke greens into the oil (with bacon, if using).

5. Add salt, pepper, and smoked paprika.

6. Sauté for 10 minutes and serve with hot sauce, and cider and vinegar, if using.

Some people in the South love to add scrambled eggs to this dish. I prefer eating mine with beans and cornbread.

GOLDENROD AND NETTLES: NOT EXACTLY YOUR GRANNY'S CORNBREAD

I omit the sugar because I do not love sweet cornbread. For vegans, substitute the eggs with a vegan mayonnaise—¼ cup is the equivalent of 1 egg. Substitute the buttermilk with 1 cup nondairy milk mixed with 1 tablespoon lemon juice, apple cider vinegar, or white vinegar.

½ cup butter, melted

2 large eggs

1 cup buttermilk

⅔ cup white sugar, maple syrup, or raw sugar

1 cup cornmeal

1 cup self-rising flour

¼ cup fresh or dried nettles or small handful (optional)

¼ cup dry or ½ cup fresh goldenrod (if fresh, well chopped; remove stems, just use leaf and flowers; optional)

1. Preheat the oven to 400°F and then add butter to a cast iron skillet; place in the oven for approximately 5 minutes until the butter is melted, then remove the skillet from the oven.

2. While the skillet is heating, combine the eggs and buttermilk (or the vegan substitutes) in a bowl until blended.

3. In a separate bowl, whisk together the sugar, cornmeal, and flour.

4. Combine the dry and wet ingredients, then add the nettles and goldenrod. Pour in the hot butter that you heated in the skillet.

5. Stir all the ingredients until well blended and few lumps remain.

6. Coat your skillet with the butter remaining in the skillet or spray on cooking spray (this ensures that the cornbread will not stick to the skillet after baking). Then add the cornmeal batter to the pan.

7. Bake in the preheated oven for 30 to 45 minutes, or until a toothpick inserted in the center of the cornbread comes out clean.

8. Remove the skillet from the oven and allow the cornbread to cool for about 15 minutes and prepare for the grand flip.

9. Loosen the cornbread around the sides in the skillet with a butter knife.

10. Place a plate on top of the skillet and, holding the plate gently, turn over the skillet and you have a piece of crispy heaven on a plate!

FRIED DANDELION FLOWER FRITTERS

2 cups dandelion flowers removing the green stem

1 cup all–purpose flour

1 cup fine corn meal

salt and pepper, to taste

¼ cup dried nettles or ½ cup fresh nettles leaves finely chopped (optional)

¼ teaspoon vitex (optional)

½ to 1 tablespoon creole seasoning (optional)

diced, deseeded jalapeno pepper, to taste (optional)

¼ cup milk or vegan milk

1 egg

½ cup oil, or enough to coat 1 inch of pan

1. Start with harvesting your dandelion blossoms from an area that has not been sprayed with pesticides. Make sure you remove the stem and green parts, which give a bitter taste.

2. Gently rinse off your flowers under cool water and pat them dry with paper towels. Set them aside while you make the batter. You can save the dandelion leaves to sauté them or you can make a quick salad with them as a side dish. If you have an abundance of dandelions, you can also make a beautiful cordial by packing the flowers into a mason jar, adding sliced lemons and sugar, and covering the mixture with vodka or gin and letting it sit for 4 to 6 weeks.

3. In a medium bowl, combine 1 cup of all-purpose flour, 1 cup of fine cornmeal, salt to taste, and black pepper to taste. No one likes a boring batter, so get creative! You can add fresh herbs from your garden or dried herbs like oregano, parsley, basil, vitex, and nettles, or even add my creole seasoning (see page 124).

4. For an extra kick, add in jalapeno pepper (optional).

5. Add ¼ cup of milk to make a creamy, wet batter, and mix well.

6. Crack and whisk in 1 large egg (I add in a few dashes of hot sauce).

7. Fold in 2 cups of the dandelion flowers into the batter mixture.

8. Add 1 inch of oil to a hot cast iron skillet.

9. Scoop a tablespoon of the mixture. Working in small batches and making sure not to put too many or crowd the pan, fry the fritters in 1 inch of oil until crispy and golden brown. This takes about 5 minutes. Remove the fritters with a slotted spoon and place the deep-fried dandelion fritter onto a plate lined with paper towels to remove the excess oil.

10. Serve with an aioli (mix mayonnaise, hot sauce, ¼ teaspoon horseradish, 3 crushed or minced garlic cloves, peeled and minced, lemon juice, salt, and pepper).

GRANNY'S BISCUITS AND GRAVY, VEGAN VERSION

1 tablespoon apple cider vinegar

1 cup nondairy milk

2 cups unbleached all-purpose flour, plus more for dusting

1 tablespoon baking powder

½ teaspoon baking soda

¾ teaspoon sea salt

4 tablespoons cold nondairy, unsalted butter, plus extra for brushing to tops of the biscuits

1. Preheat the oven to 450°F and add apple cider vinegar to nondairy milk to make "vegan buttermilk." Set aside.

2. In a large mixing bowl, whisk together the dry ingredients.

3. Add the cold butter and use your finger as a pastry cutter, or two forks, to combine the butter and dry ingredients until only small pieces remain and the mixture looks like sand. Work quickly so the butter does not get too warm.

4. Make a well in the dry ingredients and, using a wooden spoon, stir gently while pouring in the vegan "buttermilk," ¼ cup at a time. You may not need all of it. Stir the mixture until just combined and stop when the mixture resembles a slightly tacky but moldable dough.

5. Turn the dough onto a lightly floured surface, dust the top with a bit of flour, and then very gently turn the dough over on itself 5 to 6 times, lightly kneading it. Add more flour, as needed, to prevent sticking.

6. Form the dough into a 1-inch-thick disk, handling it as little as possible.

7. Use a cookie cutter or a similarly shaped object with sharp edges (such as a cocktail shaker or a small wide-mouth mason jar) and push straight down through the dough, then twist slightly. Gently reform the dough and cut out several more biscuits—you should have 7 to 8 biscuits. Grease a baking sheet with butter or line it with parchment paper; place the biscuits in two rows, making sure they just touch—this will help them rise uniformly.

8. Melt the remaining nondairy butter and brush the tops of the biscuits with it (tip: you can gently press a small divot into the center of each biscuit by using two fingers). This will also help them rise evenly, so the middle will not form a dome.

9. Bake for 10 to 15 minutes, or until the biscuits are fluffy and slightly golden brown. Serve immediately.

Tips: Pick a good playlist to dance to. I listen to the blues!

HERBED VEGAN SAUSAGE GRAVY

olive oil

vegan sausage of choice, crumbled (can substitute sautéed mushrooms and onions)

3 tablespoons vegan butter

4 tablespoons chickpea, rice, or all-purpose flour

salt and pepper, to taste

½ teaspoon poultry seasoning

4 to 5 leaves fresh (chopped fine) or ½ teaspoon dried sage

2 pinches vitex powder (optional)

3 cups vegan milk of choice (may need more if mixture is too thick)

~~~~~~~~~~

1. Add the oil to the pan and fry the crumbled sausage; remove the sausage from the pan and put it aside.

2. Add the butter and 1 tablespoon of the olive oil to the pan.

3. Add the flour and blend together with the seasonings to make the roux.

4. Slowly pour in the milk, a little at a time, while whisking the mixture vigorously (you do not want lumpy gravy).

5. Keep whisking until the roux begins to boil slightly and thickens; then add the sausage.

6. Reduce heat to a simmer and let the roux thicken.

LEMON BALM DROP BISCUITS

1 cup vegan milk

1 cup lemon balm, tightly packed (1.5 ounces by weight)

2 cups unbleached, all-purpose flour

1 tablespoon baking powder

2 pinches ginger

2 pinches cinnamon

2 tablespoons sugar (can add more depending on how sweet you want your biscuits)

1 pinch American ginseng (optional)

⅓ cup salted, cold vegan butter (I prefer Miyoko's)

Key Lime Honey Butter

2 tablespoons salted vegan butter

½ teaspoon honey (omit if vegan)

zest of 2 key limes or half a lime's worth of zest

2 droppers mimosa elixir (optional)

~~~~~~~~~

1. Preheat the oven to 425°F. Line a baking sheet with parchment paper or a silicone baking mat.

2. In a blender, combine the milk and lemon balm. Puree. Set aside.

3. In a large bowl, whisk together the flour, baking powder, ginger, cinnamon, sugar, and ginseng, if using.

4. Add the cold butter to the flour mixture and, using a pastry blender or fingers, mix together until the mixture resembles coarse cornmeal.

5. Pour in the milk mixture and stir together until well combined.

6. Drop the batter by large tablespoonfuls onto a baking sheet, about 3 inches apart.

7. Bake in a preheated oven for 12 to 15 minutes or until lightly browned.

8. To make the honey butter: While your biscuits are baking, add the vegan butter, honey, mimosa elixir, and lime zest into a small bowl. Whip until mixed. Then smother the biscuits in that honey butter.

TIPS

Fresh lemon balm works best, but if all you have is dried, let it sit in milk for 15 minutes to absorb as much liquid as it takes to release flavor.

You can substitute for lemon balm other herbs like nettles, roses, or any one of your favorites.

You can substitute the honey with butter for a vegan option.

You might as well make some cheesy, garlicky, vegan nettles biscuits for breakfast. I used the same recipe as my lemon balm biscuits. Here are my variations ... you just have to make the vegan sausage gravy.

* Omit the sugar and lemon balm.
* Add ½ cup of dried nettles to the almond milk with some minced garlic, then blend the mixture.
* Add in poultry seasoning (½ teaspoon) and powdered garlic (2 teaspoons) to the flour mixture.
* Add ½ cup vegan cheese.
* Make a garlic butter "drip" by melting butter and adding fresh minced garlic or garlic powder.

LUCRETIA'S KICKIN' CREOLE SEASONING

I am into making my own spice blends lately; that way I can also add more plant medicine. Most commercial blends include too much salt. Making spice blends gives me a chance to add more love and plant medicine to them.

I like my seasoning spicy, but you can omit the cayenne or add it to taste. Use dried or fresh thyme or oregano (either spicy or regular) from your garden.

1 part = 1 tablespoon

2 parts smoked paprika	1 part onion powder
2 parts regular paprika	½ part fresh oregano
½ part black pepper	½ part fresh thyme
½ part white pepper	¼ part nettles powder
2 to 3 heavy pinches cayenne	¼ part vitex powder
2 parts roasted and/or regular garlic powder	

1. Put all the ingredients into a blender or your NutriBullet and pulse until well blended.

2. Add salt as needed in your cooking.

Grits

I have not met a grits dish I didn't like. I mean, I am truly Southern, and my house will never be without them. According to some old tales of the South, when a woman is making you a good pot of grits, she is looking for a marriage proposal. My cousin makes the most amazing grits: We actually nicknamed them the "sexy grits" because they make you "sang" when you eat them. She was my inspiration to really get good at my grits game!

We do not believe in instant grits in the South. To make the recipe I provide, prepare to spend a good 30 minutes stirring. You might as well put some prayers and love in there. It is an ancestor connection. It is said for recipes that you sprinkle until the ancestor says, "Stop child!" Pinches of salt (magic and medicinal properties of purification and protection), sprinkles of pepper, pats of butter, and always (at least in my world, some vegan milk to get the real creaminess).

The great debates of grits: cheese or no cheese.

The greatest debate that will divide a family is salt and pepper, or sugar.

If you want to really get a heated discussion, mention this to anyone in the South. You are either strong one way or the other. I am a firm NO SUGAR!

In the South we always talk about food. We can be talking about the next meal while eating another. One night at a dinner party, a friend told a story of her father and the previous holiday, when the family discovered he was a secret sugar grits person. His mom/her grandmother were flabbergasted, and they ended up having an hour of heated discussion. The only thing that stopped it was that dessert was served. The alchemy of grits is a beautiful thing. Here is how to cook an amazing pot of love. Many suppliers of grits and rice credit Black farmers for being the reason we still have heirloom seeds and for continuing the legacy of these grains.

GRITS WITH GREENS

1 cup white or yellow grits

4 cups water

1½ teaspoons salt and pepper, or to taste

4 tablespoons unsalted butter

½ cup finely chopped kale, fresh nettles, dandelion greens, moringa, and/or collard greens (or ¼ cup dried nettles); I love to use a combination of greens.

1. Combine the grits, water, salt, pepper, and 4 tablespoons of butter in a large saucepan and bring to a boil.

2. Reduce the heat to low, cover the pan, and simmer, stirring occasionally, until the mixture is tender, about 30 minutes. If the grits become too thick, add more water or your favorite milk for a creamier texture.

✿ I sometimes add a handful of finely chopped kale, dandelion, or other greens during the cooking.

3. Complete your grits experience and top with sautéed shrimp, crumbled vegetarian sausage, cheese, or sautéed greens, or create a grits bowl bar!

VEGAN OKRA STEW

Okra stew is a staple of many parts of Africa, including Nigeria, Ghana, and Cameroon. It is made in various ways using smoked turkey wings, cow's feet, fish, shrimp, oxtails, beef, pork, and even goat meat. This is my vegan version, inspired by recipes of the Motherland. It is full of flavor, but feel free to add your favorite meat to it and make it your own. Okra has a beautiful, rich history in Africa and has many nutritional properties. I have become more obsessed with this jewel, thinking back to how okra traveled to the New World along with Africans. I am finding every way possible to add it into my diet in a form other than the fried version I grew up on. It is a staple in Louisiana, where it is used in gumbo.

I love to cook dried black-eyed peas and use the leftovers in this dish the next day. For the broth, you can also use bone or medical mushroom broth.

2 tablespoons olive or palm oil (you can use your herbal-infused oil mentioned in Chapter 5)

1 medium onion, peeled, diced, and sautéed

1 green or red pepper, seeded, diced, and sautéed

1 to 2 cups thinly sliced fresh collard greens, moringa leaves, spinach, or swiss chard

4 to 6 cloves garlic, peeled and minced

2 (14.5-ounce) cans fire-roasted diced tomatoes

1 (6-ounce) can tomato paste

½ pound okra, rinsed and sliced in half or left whole with ends cut

1 small 10-ounce bag frozen corn

1 small bag frozen or 1 (15.5-ounce) can black-eyed peas, drained

1 to 2 pinches cayenne, for extra heat

salt and pepper, to taste

1 bay leaf

2 tablespoons creole seasoning (see page 124)

handful chopped fresh or dried nettles, destemmed

1 container vegetable, chicken, or beef stock

~~~~~~~~~~~~~

1. In a medium pot, add the oil, onion, pepper, collards, and garlic, and sauté until softened.

2. Add the tomatoes, tomato paste, okra, corn, and black-eyed peas and stir the mixture.

3. Add the spices and nettles, and stir the mixture, adding more spices to taste.

4. Add stock or broth and stir until mixed; cover the pot and reduce the heat to a simmer and cook for 45 minutes.

5. Serve alone, over rice, with cornbread, or with fufu (doughlike fufu is made from boiled and pounded starchy foods like plantains, cassava, and yams).

My dear teacher Sobonfu Some' said a house without an altar is ungrounded. I spent time with her and learned her lessons of honoring those who have transitioned from their physical bodies. This was very important in deepening my understanding of grief; I missed those loved ones and had reverence for those who helped me create ways to keep memories of them alive in my daily practice. That is what canning and cooking are to me—honoring traditions that have been passed down in my family for generations. All of us have a connection to the plants and food preservation in our DNA; if we didn't, we wouldn't be here.

Since the beginning of time, the need to store food has been very important for survival. I remember from my youth the outline of an old Spring House, a shack built over a creek that would act as the refrigerator when my grandpa was young on the farm.

I also have memories of the place under my grandparents' house, below the sun porch, that was used as a root cellar. I would have to climb under there and bring out potatoes and other root vegetables. The smell of dirt on potatoes still brings back those memories.

Shelves of mason jars were full of love and the bountiful harvest of the season. The cement building behind the garage was a meat storage area for hanging meats from the farms of family members and our own. I did not know the importance of these converted spaces until I was much older. Because food was always plentiful, I also did not realize that my family was not rich.

The amazing Leah Penniman, who wrote *Farming While Black,* is a food and social justice advocate from Soul Fire Farm. She says that "to free ourselves, we must feed ourselves." In these times, we now see how the practices of those before us are more important in moving forward.

Canning was a community practice in my youth. It was a way for our family to honor the land and feed ourselves in the winter months. So much is lost when we do not connect with the community. Some' always talked about her African village in Burkina Faso and how everything was done in the community. Known for her grief rituals, she spoke about the importance of joining together for healing and the higher purpose of the community. It made me realize how far we have strayed from the old ways. In her tradition—that of the West African Dagara tribe—according to the Dagara Cosmology Wheel,[32] each person has a specific role based on their elemental nature. You find yours by the last number of your birth year: fire (two and seven), water (one and six), nature (three and eight), earth (zero and five), and mineral (four and

32 Malidoma Patrice Somé, *The Healing Wisdom of Africa: Finding Life Purpose through Nature, Ritual, and Community* (TarcherPerigeen, 1999). Also see a speech given by Malidoma in 1995 on the basics of Dagara Cosmology: http://archive.constantcontact.com /fs012/1101454195791/archive/1104070256872.html and "The Seen and the Unseen," by Sobonfu Somé: https://www.culturalsurvival.org/publications/cultural-survival -quarterly/seen-and-unseen-spirituality-among-dagara-people.

nine). Each has a characteristic purpose for how people relate and how to maintain the balance of the village. It is easy to create community circles for herbal medicine and food preservation. Find a friend who has a friend and so on. Explore your elemental nature for your family and your circle to see how to better support one another.

Connecting to our ancestors by using plants from our native lands helps intensify our magic. If you have living relatives, ask questions about your roots and homeland. Do they remember any herbal medicines used in the family? If you know where your family is from, research the plant medicine of the area.

Magical Canning Recipes with Herbs

FIRE CIDER SWEET HEAT PICKLES

Prepare fire cider with the recipe on page 111.

4 cups thickly sliced pickling cucumbers (8 to 10 pickling cucumbers)

1 cup peeled and sliced onion (about 1 large)

2 tablespoons pickling salt

1 cup apple cider vinegar or fire cider

¾ cup granulated sugar

4 tablespoons pickling spice

½ teaspoon red pepper flakes

1 cayenne pepper, chopped for extra heat

love as the final ingredient

1. Wash 2 pint-size jars or a large pot for 15 minutes to sanitize, or use your dishwasher to skip this step. Combine the sliced cucumbers, onion, and pickling salt in a colander set in a large bowl. Refrigerate for 1 hour to remove excess liquid. Rinse the vegetables well and discard the liquid.

2. Combine the vinegar or fire cider and sugar in a large pot. Heat over medium heat until the sugar is dissolved. Add the pickling spice, red

pepper flakes, and chopped cayenne pepper. Increase the heat to high and bring the brine to a boil.

3. Add the drained vegetables and stir to combine. Cook for 5 minutes or until all the vegetables in the brine are fully heated through. Using tongs, fill the sterilized jars with the vegetables. Slowly pour the hot brine over the vegetables in each jar, leaving ½ inch headspace.

4. Gently tap the jars on a towel-lined countertop to help loosen any bubbles before using a wooden chopstick to dislodge any remaining bubbles. Check the headspace again and add more brine if necessary.

5. Wipe the rims, apply the lids and rings, and process in a hot-water bath for 10 minutes.

6. Let these pickles cure on the counter for 48 hours to 14 days before eating. Remember to label the jars with the date!

SPICED PEACH PIE JAM WITH SELF-HEAL HERBAL INFUSION

Self-Heal *(Prunella vulgaris)*—prepare this herbal infusion before beginning the process. Put a small handful of dried or chopped fresh self-heal herb (also called heal-all) in a mason jar, fill with boiling water, cover, and allow it to sit for 2 to 4 hours. Strain and use this herbal infusion with peaches. It adds the beautiful magic of healing oneself with each bite. This recipe makes a great pie filling too.

Yield: About 6 half-pint jars

3¾ cups chopped peaches (about 3 pounds)

¼ cup lemon juice

½ teaspoon cinnamon

¼ teaspoon nutmeg

1 teaspoon vanilla extract

1 package powdered pectin (I like Sure Jell brand)

5 cups sugar

½ cup Self-Heal herbal infusion (optional)

1. Sterilize canning jars and prepare two-piece canning lids according to the manufacturer's directions.

2. To prepare fruit: Sort and wash fully ripe peaches. Remove the stems, skins, and pits. Crush the peaches.

3. A tip about processing peaches is to slice an "X" onto the top of each peach and dip them into boiling water. Let them sit for 3 minutes and carefully remove them from the water; let them cool slightly, making sure not to burn yourself; skins should slide off easily.

4. To make the jam: Measure chopped peaches into a heavy-bottomed pot. Add the lemon juice, spices, vanilla, Self-Heal herbal infusion, and pectin; stir well. Place on high heat and, stirring constantly; bring quickly to a full boil with bubbles over the entire surface. Add the sugar, continue stirring, and heat again to full boil. Boil hard for 1 minute, stirring constantly. Remove from the heat and skim off the foam.

5. Put the hot jam immediately into hot, sterile jars, leaving ¼-inch head-space. Wipe the rims of the jars with a dampened, clean paper towel; adjust the 2-piece metal canning lids. Process in a boiling water canner pot for 10 to 15 minutes (see note below for times according to jar size).

SAVORY PEACH PRESERVES WITH DETOXIFYING CHAI SPICE

This is similar to a chutney or tomato jam with a twist on an old flavor; plus during peach season, you have to get creative with all these amazing peaches in the South.

5 large peaches

½ cup rice wine vinegar or apple cider vinegar

½ cup sugar (coconut, date, honey, or any sweetener alternative will do)

your favorite chai tea blend

If you don't have chai tea, you can use these herbs and spices:

1 teaspoon coriander seed

1 teaspoon black peppercorn

3 to 4 cardamom pods

1 teaspoon clove

3 bay leaves

1 tablespoon nettle

1 (3-inch) dried or fresh dandelion root, chopped fine

cinnamon

1 to 2 red chiles (pinch of cayenne or red pepper flakes, to taste; you can omit if you do not like the heat)

1. Roughly chop the peaches. Put them in a pot.

2. Add in the remaining ingredients, cover the pot, and cook on medium-high heat for 5 to 7 minutes until the peaches soften; stir the mixture often.

3. Lower heat to a simmer and cook for 25 minutes. Watch it so it does not burn.

4. Ladle into jars; it will keep in the fridge for 1 month.

LOVE JAM

This recipe is inspired by my love for plants, especially those who help heal the sacred heart space. I harvested the ones I used while spending the afternoon with my beloved friend's toddler. All the best harvests are done surrounded by love.

If I have one goal, it is to leave a legacy of self-love to everyone I meet. This recipe is a physical embodiment of that. Muscadine is my grandmother's pure love for me, and it is also the first jelly I learned to make. In the South we are blessed with these little muscadine jewels. Snacking on them while running around my grandparents' farm was my childhood.

Muscadines are high in antioxidants, even more so than blueberries and pomegranates.

Ashley Cobb, clinical dietitian at WakeMed hospitals, has this to say about muscadines, which are especially high in the antioxidants resveratrol and ellagic acid.

"Resveratrol is an antioxidant that is responsible for red wine's heart-healthy reputation, ... and the mighty muscadine has nine times more antioxidant power than red grapes used to make California's red wines. They also contain six times the fiber, and muscadine wines may contain three to four times the number of phenolic compounds (which have antioxidant properties), plus a higher ellagic acid content than your average red wine.

Resveratrol helps to decrease cholesterol, fight cancer, and some newer studies show that it may reduce the risk of age-related diseases such as Alzheimer's, cardiovascular disease, high—blood pressure, Crohn's, Parkinson's, and more, and ultimately may lengthen one's lifespan. ... Ellagic acid is another type of antioxidant that is being investigated in cancer prevention research ... Muscadines are also fat—free, high in fiber, low in sodium and an excellent source of manganese."[33]

The jelly-making and canning processes are so special to me. My grandmother transitioned to being an ancestor (she died) when I was in my early twenties. I was broken and went far from the life I had and did everything wrong in the grieving process. Now these herbs and canning have been such an important ritual in my healing process, not to mention a useful skill in these modern times. It brings her home to my heart and soul. While making the traditional recipe, I thought, What if I brought the plants in more? I might as well add a flower and crystal essence and a tincture too. How much love can you put in one jar? Let's do this! I won an award for this recipe at the International Herb Symposium and it was a last-minute entry five minutes before closing. It was the first time I had submitted an entry to an herbal competition. When I

33 https://www.wakemed.org/mighty-muscadines.

won, I instantly thought of my ancestors and felt them celebrating with me. It was not a huge award but it was very important for me and a way to honor the old ways and my ancestors.

3 cups freshly picked violet flowers, loosely packed (optional)

handful dried red rose petals

handful tulsi (holy basil)

½ handful lemon balm

3 cups muscadine juice (see recipe on page 137) or store-bought concord grape juice

3 cups apple juice

3 cups sugar (I prefer raw sugar or turbinado sugar)

1 pink box low-sugar pectin

1. Place the violets, rose petals, tulsi, and lemon balm into a quart mason jar.

2. Pour the muscadine juice into the herbal mixture and let it sit for 1 to 3 hours to infuse (longer time equals more flavor).

3. Add the apple juice (which has a high level of pectin and assists in jelling when you use less sugar).

4. Check exact measurements for final liquid total: 6 cups total of juices and infusion.

5. Add the liquid into heavy-bottomed pot.

6. Add the sugar to the mixture and bring it to a slight boil, melting all the sugar.

7. Add the pectin (if using regular pectin instead of the lower-sugar version, follow the recipe exactly as listed on the box in order to use the correct amount of sugar).

8. Turn up the heat until you get a steady boil, even when you stir the mixture.

9. Stir constantly until the magical process of jellying occurs (the mixture will thicken and coat the back of the spoon when done).

10. I like to stir in a few dried crushed rose petals at the end.

11. Ladle the jelly into jars, leaving ½ inch headspace.

12. Wipe the glass jars clean and then attach the metal lids.

13. Gently place the jars into a large pot of boiling water, one jar at a time, and make sure the water completely covers them; let them sit for 10 minutes.

14. Have on hand a folded towel or solid surface, like a cutting board on which to cool the jars. You should start to hear a light "ping" or "pop"— these sounds let you know that the jars have sealed properly. I get excited when I hear those sounds!

TIPS

* **Washing:** Prewash the jelly jars and boil them to sanitize them before you use them. I sometimes put them in the dishwasher to do both.

* **Timing the water-bath method for sealing jars:** Bring water that covers the jars to a rolling boil, and then cover the canner and boil for 10 minutes if you are using 4-, 8-, or 12-ounce jars, or for 15 minutes if you are using 16-ounce jars. Check individual jelly/preserves recipes for more specific processing times.

Herb Knowledge

The rose is good for circulation and one of the best spiritual energetics in most heart-healing formulas.

Holy basil, a.k.a. vana tulsi, is a great tonic for balancing the body and provides great emotional support, especially for people dealing with PTSD, tension, or underlying fear. Considered a sacred plant in households in India, holy basil has brought much joy to my life. Vana tulsi (*Ocimum* gratiss*imum*), native to East Africa, has a large quantity of euganol (oil of clove).

Harvesting violet flowers can be meditative. It takes time to gather them so find a great song to sing and dream of childhood days when these simple tasks brought hours of entertainment.

Extra love: Add a dropper full of grief tincture, such as blends of mimosa, hawthorn, or lemon balm.

Flower essence of okra is a deeply spiritual plant to many African people. The vegetable has numerous health benefits. Spiritually, the plant energy works on the lower chakras, which are power centers, by "moving" stuck energy.

MUSCADINE JUICE

3 cups water or enough
to cover the grapes

2 pounds muscadine grapes

1. Boil the grapes until you see them break down, approximately 30 minutes, mashing them occasionally with a potato masher.

2. Strain the mixture by allowing it to sit in a fine sieve over a heat-proof bowl and letting gravity drain the liquid out of the grapes; then strain the mixture in a cheesecloth and carefully pour the hot grape juice in a mason jar.

Note: You can skip this step of making your own juice and instead buy a 64-ounce container of Concord grape juice (use 3 cups), or you can omit the apple juice and use 6 cups of the grape juice.

Do you want to learn more about canning? Enjoy this resource from the National Center for Home Food Preservation, https://nchfp.uga .edu.

CHAPTER 7

CEREMONIES FOR SELF-TRANSFORMATION

I often joke that I was an alchemist in utero and that the only reason I am here today is through my lifelong practice of creating ceremonies for myself and the plants that helped me heal. As a child I would mix roots, red dirt, and flowers down by the creek on my grandparents' farm. I would recite prayers to God and nature or just to thank the land. I did not know that it was a practice till my first time visiting Beaufort, South Carolina, which is a chain of islands where my stepfather's people are from. His mother whispered in my ear when we crossed through a certain island, telling me this was where they practiced hoodoo, and some people called them root workers.

She said, "See the houses and how they have the dark paint outlining the doors and windows; that is to keep the evil spirits out." She also told me how there were people you would see who helped you with your problems. They made charm bags and other things to protect you, she said. Some of them could hurt people but, mostly, they were there to work magic to help you get what you needed or desired. When I heard this, I was so in awe. I remember thinking that I hoped I could meet one of them or do those things myself one day. Although my stepdad's mother was white, she was the first person who showed no fear for what had been a part of me and other African Americans of the South all my life. It gave me hope that there were others who saw the world and its magic like I did. I realized early that white traditions were different from Black traditions, and I was beginning to see how to bridge the two worlds.

She was also the first person who took me to a Church of God, where I heard folks speaking in tongues and saw the minister "laying hands" (some call it Reiki) on people. The service was loud and not what I was used to growing up Southern Baptist. I thought to myself, I want to do that when I am older. I did not know what "that" was exactly, but I did know that it was my destiny. Later in my teenage years I met a woman who worked in a movie rental store and who looked at me and said, "I hope you know what you are." She was saying that I was a medicine woman—or witch, as some people say.

I began to learn about ceremonies of witchcraft because I knew I was "different." But then, I knew there were others "like me." My tiny town had only four or five books in the library on witchcraft—that's it.

Slowly, through the adventures I had while I was growing up and continuing to practice, I found my way home to my African roots, our traditions, and to a connection with the elements. My ancestors were calling me, and they brought me back because I did not know there was a name for what I was.

Rootworkers have always been important in the healing arts in the South. Often viewed as part doctor, part priest, and workers of the plants, they were the inheritors of the practices that so many of our ancestors brought with them from Africa and the Caribbean, practices that had to be hidden from the enslavers.

Walking in the Path of the Rootworker

I interviewed Ikeoma Divine, one of my favorite teachers and colleagues of rootwork, who I met while I was teaching at an herbal conference. We formed an instant bond, and I was excited to meet someone who was following a similar path. Ikeoma is a registered nurse who comes from a line of midwives, nurses, and herbalists on both sides of her family. Helping others heal has always been a passion of hers. She believes it is important to carry on this legacy both in and out of an institutional setting.

Ikeoma Divine

What is hoodoo? Does it differ from rootwork?

My name is Ikeoma Divine. Ikeoma is Igbo (Nigerian). It means "good strength." I was born in Virginia (Tidewater area), where there were a lot of Igbo people who were brought to Virginia. This name was given to me by fellow Igbo friends years ago. Hoodoo has been described as a religion. That has not been my experience. This practice has continued its legacy under the guise of Christianity. I am definitely a product of the South. Born in Virginia, raised in Louisiana and Texas, and grandparents from North and South Carolina, Georgia, and Alabama.

What I noticed as a child was that these terms hoodoo, rootwork, juju, etc., were used interchangeably in conversations, depending on where you were. The people who actually practiced it refused to admit it. It was always deemed "evil" and was definitely used to ostracize anyone from the community. At the same time, it was prevalent. It was hidden in plain sight. In any religion there are set rules for rituals. In every church service I experienced, we began with worship and praise service before the sermon. I did not see any consistency in the way people

AFRICAN AMERICAN HERBALISM

practiced. The rituals were as diverse as cornbread and potato salad recipes throughout the South. I call what I do rootwork. It is alchemy, rituals, and mediumship used for specific purposes. This is definitely an inherited practice. I tried to run away from this in my teens and twenties. When it was time for me to practice, I was called.

In your own words, how have we been able to keep these traditions?

This practice is incorporated in my life. It is not a religion for me but a spiritual journey. A journey that has transformed me, healed me, and allowed me to rediscover my life purposes. Over the years, my rituals have evolved.

What is it that you would like people to know about this craft and practice?

This is a practice of inheritance. If one is drawn to it, it's usually because they have an ancestral lineage connected to this.

How did your upbringing influence your work as a hoodoo practitioner?

I grew up in a Pentecostal Holiness Church in Louisiana in the '70s and '80s. It was there that I learned that my mediumship gift had a name, "The gift of discernment." I learned at a very young age how things were done behind closed doors. It did not all make sense until I started traveling internationally and experienced similar practices in other practices in Haiti, Ghana, Brazil, and South Africa. The similarities were a reminder that the spiritual connections were not lost. We just incorporated them under the guise of Christianity. I am glad to see how the younger generations are openly practicing the spirituality of their ancestors. They hid who they were so that we could be here and did not have to hide.

What does honoring your ancestors mean to you?

Honoring your ancestors and connecting with them is the root of this practice. Once one is able to connect, and learn to listen, the journey will begin. Always start with an ancestral altar. You will find that some of your teachers won't be in physical form.

Contact information:

Facebook, Instagram, and Twitter: @IkeomaDivine
www.ikeomaseye.com

I found out more as I began my studies of Mother Catherine Seals as well as Mother Leafy Anderson of the Spiritual church movement in New Orleans at the height of the Jim Crow era. I say Mother Catherine's spirit brought me there to heal after my "divorce" in 2020, and boy did the energy of that beautiful city and her people do that.

I visited the sites of these old churches and started interviewing a few of the elders on the "old" blending with the "new" in spirituality and the church, and it has been eye opening in so many ways. A thin line exists where our old ways blended with these new ways, hidden in plain sight.

I attended one of these services and witnessed for myself the abundance rituals, with the offering plate being passed around, the Florida water on the pulpit, and the elaborate altars all around. I have never felt church like that, so full of love. I also have felt the juju (energy) that still exists in the old home of the voodoo queen herself, Marie Laveau, when I got the honor of tending the altar there on Saint Ann Street in New Orleans French Quarter.

I also saw how in blending the Catholic saints with the orishas in Santeria, the people were still able to practice the old ways with the new, and not be punished. Elaborate ancestors' altars of the old became pictures on the wall in certain places in the home, honoring those who had passed on.

The South has its own rootwork vibe because of this blending of old and new. There was a Dr. Buzzard, a well-known rootworker whose name was Stephany Robinson. He was an African American from the island of Saint Helena (a British possession in the southern Atlantic Ocean), who began practicing rootwork in the early 1900s. He attracted clients, both locally and from around the country, until his death in early 1947. According to oral history, Robinson's father was a "witch doctor" who had been brought directly to the island of Saint Helena (then a British possession) from West Africa, despite the British ban on the importation of enslaved people from Africa. He was said to have enormous spiritual power, which he passed on to his son. Robinson was very sought after, especially in court cases where he believed that if you chewed on a certain root, you could conjure what outcome you needed. Phrases popular to the South are having the ability to "talk the fire out," which means praying to remove pain from a person. Rootwork is so deep in the culture that most people do not even realize that they too are practicing it.

Some people may say that there are only certain ways to practice, but I do not believe that about hoodoo or rootwork. It is personal to you, whom you study with, and your connection to the plants and your ancestors. In these times, people are now more fascinated with ritual and ceremonies. I am so excited to see that interest in the old ways is rising.

In this chapter, I have included ceremonies or rituals for self-transformation, protections, and other needs. I believe these practices do not have to be elaborate; when you connect with the elemental natures, your ancestors, and yourself, you become the altar and how you live becomes the ceremony. You do not need all the things out there on the market. Trust your own intuition, ask around, ask questions before receiving services, and be leery of buying things from people you do not know or whose work you do not know. Not everyone has your best intentions in mind.

Crafting Personal Ceremonies to Heal

Here are simple ways that rootwork can be used for personal transformation and protection. Rituals and ceremonies do not need to be elaborate! I have conjured more for myself by taking offerings I have picked up on walks to the riverside and praying than by using all the expensive things I have ever bought.

I have tested my practice all my life and at each rock bottom I have crossed through—such as in this past year when I had to leave my home after my seven-year relationship ended and I had to disassemble all my altars and put them in storage. I am a living embodiment of what I teach and preach, and know these things work with the help of the plants and your ancestors.

My own healing was made possible by going back to my childhood roots of plants, nature, my ancestors, rivers like the Mississippi in New Orleans and the French Broad in Asheville, North Carolina, intent, and the power of my breath with prayer. Take these practices and make them your own to lead you to your own healing and self-transformation.

Ancestor Reverence

Honoring your ancestors is an old practice very important to all indigenous cultures. If you do not honor the ones before you and know where you come from, how can you move forward?

Ancestor reverence, simply put, is creating spaces to connect with your ancestors. Create a list of the names of your ancestors, some whom you have fond memories of. Begin the morning or when you cook a meal by saying some of these names, and pray and give gratitude. You can call on the power of the ancestors when you need it. Their DNA is inside you.

Ancestor Root-Grounding Meditation

In a seated or standing position, place both feet on the floor.

Imagine your legs are like deep tree roots connecting you to the earth.

Take a deep breath while filling up the abdomen or lower belly with air. Imagine it as an inflated balloon.

With each inhale, imagine the love of your ancestors coming in.

With each exhale, imagine your love going out to them like a warm embrace.

With each inhale, imagine the love of mother earth coming up.

With each exhale, imagine your love for her spreading across the globe.

With each inhale, imagine things no longer serving you coming up.

With each exhale, imagine passing things that no longer serve you to your ancestors and these ancestors taking them from you. They want you to find joy!

Creating Ancestor Altars

The deeper your practice gets, your altar grows and changes, I believe. As you connect and work more closely with your ancestors, they begin to let you know what they want on it as well. Have you ever had a strange craving for an old something you remember your grandmother or grandfather eating? I feel that it is them talking to us. It is important to honor our loved ones by creating meals for them by using heirloom recipes from your family that they would have eaten: snacks, vices, liquors, or drinks they loved. I love to give them part of my meals to share and talk with them. Even my morning coffee is done with the ancestors. I pour them a cup, pray, and it is a perfect way to start my day!

Decorate your sacred altar space using the elements: fire (candles); water or libations (in a vessel you change out daily with clean water); earth (a plant with dirt; I have actually dirt from my ancestral land); nature (crystals, leaves, rocks, feathers, or anything that reminds you of nature); and air (incense). You can also use pictures of loved ones who have crossed over or passed away, things that represent where your people are from. Also some ancestors require liquors and some do not. My people love moonshine but they do not love bourbon. I can tell because one seems to go way faster than the other when offerings of these liquors are made on the altar.

I work with many people who have been adopted or do not know their family. I grew up on the white side of my family and I had no pictures of my father's family, so mine started with a mask from Africa to represent his side of the family. It continued to grow while I connected to them; they brought me to places where I could slowly find photos of them. That is truly why ancestral practices are so sacred to me, and I know from experience that this works.

It is the only way both sides of my family share the same table. It has brought much healing to me and the intergenerational trauma that runs through so many people's families.

Candle Magic

Throughout history candles have been used in sacred spaces to honor the loved ones who have crossed over and the religious figures of many cultures. Some people use them for magic or to call in a specific purpose. That is why I call mine sacred intent candles.

I craft my candles for clients through divination (or readings), using information I receive. I then "dress" (use specific things that relate to what the person needs) the candle with herbs/roots, conjure oils, colors, crystals, prayers, and often music to create alchemy to be able to tell a story of a healing journey. Each time you light the candle, you are reminded of the magic you and it contain. It provides you with a moment of reflection to call in the energy you require for a specific purpose. Some hoodoo practitioners use the candle to do readings or to see how and if your candle has produced your desired intent. This practice is called candle divination, in which, depending on the spiritual practices, it is believed that a candle's flame, smoke, or wax will provide insight into the future or the situation at hand.

Capromancy: This is smoke divination—reading and deciphering the patterns of the smoke or soot left after burning a candle.

Ceromancy: This is wax divination; you drop wax into water to see what images or "symbols" show up.

Pyromancy: This involves using the flame for divination. Start by asking simple "yes" or "no" questions, asking the flame to show you what "yes" or "no" is. Sometimes "yes" will be a circle and "no" will be back and forth, much like the motion of a pendulum.

You can craft your own methods using a few simple steps mentioned in this chapter.

Choosing the Right Color

Candles come in many colors; colors have specific vibrations and frequencies representing different meanings and can be burned to use in personal ceremonies in rootwork or for your specific intention or need.

Candle magic uses the concept of color spectrum, chakras, or color therapy, because each color radiates a specific wavelength of light. Certain colors also can evoke a subconscious reaction in your brain based on your unique memories and life experiences. I use the concept of color associated with the power centers, also known as chakras.

Red: root, ancestors, personal power, survival

Orange: sacral for anything from sex, to creativity, to fertility, and to abundance, and ignites the power center that controls it

Yellow: solar plexus, sharpens intuition, converts the energy of the victim to that of a victor using the lessons from our past hurt or traumas to lead us to a new way

Green: money, success, securing a job, or sacred heart-space healing

Pink: the energetic heart space, heartbreak, calling in healing to receive the love you want, to soften oneself after the trauma dealing with the heart or grief

White: can be used for all things when no other color is available, represents the high level of consciousness and purification

Black: represents protection from evil, cutting ties with people or things that no longer serve you, protection against dark forces to neutralize negative energies sent to you or loved ones, and harnesses the power of the universe

Purple: represents the "third eye" or crown seeking to expand what it already has in your higher consciousness, working in the astral or dream world, obtaining spiritual protection

Brown: represents the earth. People who burn a brown candle seek to regain balance, find refuge from chaos, find lost items, and grow a long-lasting friendship.

Gold: represents abundance in all forms, stepping into your full power, attracting a powerful influence, focusing on their goals, aligning with your sacred purpose, and calling in all things needed for transformation

How to Work with Your Sacred Intent Candle

FOCUS on the intent of your work.

I suggest making yourself a cup of tea or a special libation.

Use Florida water or rainwater to cleanse the outside of the candle to remove anyone else's juju.

Use incense to cleanse the work area and yourself.

First slightly trim the wick; this makes the candle magic personal.

Choose herbs or conjure oils in very tiny amounts to "dress" or prep the candle for what you are working on. **Be careful not to use too much; it can become flammable and dangerous!**

Poke four holes deep into the wax in the glass candle with a poker or chopstick and drip the conjure oil into the holes in the four directions (top, bottom, left, and right).

Before lighting, hold the candle with both hands and say a personal prayer or blessing for your own healing or manifestation. I suggest that each person find a personal mantra, a prayer for what you want the candle to do, a song, or an ancestor's saying that you can recite while the candle is burning ("I am all that I am" is a suggestion for building personal power, but make it personal).

Petition Work

Words are powerful, and through them, we can transcend and transform from anything. You can write words on the candle or you can write what is called a petition, which consists of what you want to call in or release. Write your desires for yourself, your purpose, and what you want to see with your business (I love to use gold pens for my abundance work). Some people also use symbols, such as a *veve*, which is a religious symbol commonly used in different branches of vodun throughout the African diaspora.

Place the petition under or on the altar with the candle and recite the words to your candle.

Feed the energy of the candle with your sacred wishes each time you light it. When you want to call in love or abundance, fold the paper three times toward you. If you are trying to release or remove something, like a bad relationship, ill intent, or even sickness, fold it three times away from you.

Suggestion: I [list name] call in the power of my ancestors for my highest and greatest good, as well as my spirit guides to assist in this task [list what you want to achieve, release, or protect yourself from].

Burn your petition and then scatter the ashes. For me, it is either down by the riverside for abundance. For calling things in quickly, scatter them at a crossroads or intersection where that location will open the ways for it to happen. And, of course, you can always use your own yard.

TIPS

When you are "dressing" or working with your candle, such as when it is burning or when you are creating any of these ceremonial pieces for yourself, it is important for you to center yourself and focus on the energy of what you are working toward. The intent is important and it is three-quarters of the conjure energy. Each moment, our DNA is changing, and how we speak to ourselves is like downloading into the universe what we want. These moments give us time to reflect on self-talk as well, so visit your candle often.

Never leave a burning candle unattended and do not blow it out; you need to snuff out the flame.

Gris-Gris Bags

Gris-gris bags are personal pouches, like a charm, talisman, or amulet, used in Africa or the Caribbean. Incorporated into the hoodoo or root-worker traditions, they contain herbs and other articles. Gris-gris bags, typically carried on the body, are used for protection, luck, abundance, or anything else you may need.

High John the Conqueror root, used for luck, most often appears in these bags; shells, bone, and rootwork oils also are used to personalize the bags.

Love and Healing Heartbreak

Honey Jar: This is used to bring sweetness and abundance into your life. Take a small jar and fill it with honey. Add fresh flowers, such as roses, honeysuckle, and lavender to bring in peace and ease during the process, or add things you can find in your yard or local market that speak to you. You can write out your problems or what you want to call in with love. You can put it in your altar space. I do not put the written words in the jar; I use them as a visual element or burn them and take the honey jar to the river to speak about what problems I am working with or what I want to call in. I love to make offerings of desserts or oranges. If your heart is broken, cry that out if you need to. This ceremony has brought me the most healing in my times of need.

This can also work as an abundance ritual by adding abundance herbs such as goldenrod, as well as money offerings and citrine crystal.

During this ceremony, bring some libations, like water or alcohol, to pour to honor the ancestors and spirits.

Closure ceremony: For those with a broken heart, I suggest a ceremony that requires writing a breakup letter to the person who broke your heart. This helps with closure. I believe the person does not have to be present for closure to happen; that is what the ceremony is for. The brain does not know if you are doing it with the person; the ceremony helps gets the words and emotions out. It can be combined with cord-cutting ceremonies by braiding together three white, black, or red strings, each about six inches long. Then at the end of the ceremony, read your letter out loud and use scissors to cut the cords in the middle. Burn all of this and scatter the ashes.

I also use this as a breaking-up ceremony for myself, acknowledging my own behaviors that keep me from love or abundance due to traumas. I write a letter to myself thanking those behaviors for keeping me safe and stating that I do not need them anymore. Sometimes we have a full release so that we can receive our blessings with both hands and an open heart. This closure ceremony has been so powerful for me in creating a life bigger than what I could have ever imagined!

Candles: Black, green, or pink for heart healing; gold or green for abundance; white for purifying

Herbal Suggestions to Take for Support

Mimosa: for bringing to the surface deep-seated grief; medicinally used for its mood-elevating and calming-anxiety effects

Rose: for protection while the heart heals energetically from pain

Lavender: for teaching us that healing does not have to be hard, and for adding grace to the healing journey

Damiana: for stepping into sexual power and transforming it into creativity; for invoking self-validation of your own beauty and sexuality

Calendula: for bringing in abundance on all levels of joy, money, and love

Motherwort: for calming and healing with the mother energy

Kava: for moving out ego and moving forward from a heart-centered space

Protection

Freezer spells stop ill intent from coming your way. I once had to do this for a client whose manager was harassing them and threatening to stop them from getting a promotion. I took a small jar filled with water and herbs like rue for protection, lavender for grace and ease, and mugwort to remove negative energy. I added the name of the manager to the jar, sealed it, and put it in the freezer. Later that week, my client noticed the manager just stayed away and the client's promotion came more quickly, removing that client from the manager's supervision.

I have also used rootwork to help protect a woman and her children in a domestic violence situation. No harm was done to the perpetrator; he just simply decided it was time for him to move across the country.

Railroad ties at your front door keep out unwanted negative energy. Wherever I go, this is a primary way I keep things from getting in. I also keep them in my car, and I give them to my beloved to keep them safe. Simply go to the railroad tracks and find one; also, some botanicas sell them.

Black tourmaline is a stone I place above my front and back doors as well.

Grief

"Surrendering to your sorrow has the power to heal the deepest of wounds," says Sobonfu Some'. Grief is a multilayered process, and the grief ritual is a time for community, holding space, and release. Some' comes from the Dagara tribe of Burkina Faso, and her village has a tradition that no one grieves alone. They join periodically to grieve, a practice mostly absent in Western cultures. While sharing space with her, I learned so much about grief. Often we think that grief is just about someone who has passed away, but it comes in so many more places: the loss of a relationship, job, friend, pet, or who we thought we "would be."

I believe that we can create sacred space as we journey through our bodies by using plant spirit meditation, the power of the elements, and breath work to move the grief while nourishing ourselves in these spaces.

To honor the work and the ways of my dear teacher Some', we will cocreate three altars. Bring or collect nature articles to adorn them. The first altar honors your ancestors to call in for support, using your family pictures or things that honor your ancestors. The second one is a self-love altar of things that inspire you and bring you strength. The third altar is for those who need space for a deeper release and creates a space in your home or in nature where you can go to grieve. Always call in your friends or community to "hold space"—not try to fix things but sometimes just to sit quietly with you.

Spend as much time as you can with your ancestors at the altar! Ask them for help during this time; they are always there for you, even when you feel no one else is.

Herbal Remedies for Tea and Tinctures

Mimosa: helps move deep grief

Motherwort: this plant is *Leonurus cardiaca,* which translates to "lion heart": it uses that energy to help us be bold and assist us in times of need; medicinally helps with anxiety, which makes this plant a favorite

Holy basil: great for PTSD

St. John's wort: use the oil to anoint the skin on the area around your heart and even the area around your vulva to help energetically heal sexual trauma

Rose: helps protect the heart, allowing it to bloom while being protected (think of how rose thorns help "protect" the flower so you must be gentle as you approach a rose)

Skull cap: to calm the nerves

"Fixing" candles for grief: choose white (purify), red (ancestor support or grounding), or pink (healing the energetic heart, bringing love); for a bad relationship use a black candle on a bed of salt (to cut ties with people not serving you or to create a space to actively grieve)

Spiritual bath: any of the herbs listed above

Okra: moves stagnant energy in the body

Hyssop: helps purify the energetic body

Lavender: gives us permission to have grace and gentleness during grieving and healing

Using the elements: This was an important part of the grief ritual with Sobonfu Some': visit nature often to help release and receive the energy. Rivers are my favorite for release, as are crying and prayers for healing. Go to the forest for support and grounding.

While you are there, write, scream, cry ... release.

CHAPTER 8

LIVING LEGACIES

While researching for this book, I more deeply understood that our history was passed down by oral tradition and that, unfortunately, most people are not as recognized for their work until they are gone. This chapter is dedicated to the living legacies of our ancestors, who are continuing the work. These are colleagues whose work honors their ancestor connection and culture and who are doing amazing work as herbalists to preserve the tradition. They inspire me as herbalists and healers who are working on multiple platforms and spaces, who turn toward one another. They are the ones helping the community—which is what our people do with the plants.

The world of herbalism often excludes the stories of people of color. Though our stories are complex and some are full of pain, they are the embodiment of the true essence of healing with plants and of the ways of our people before we arrived here in chains.

When I was writing and looking for resources, I found it very difficult to find writings by people of color about people of color. It was extremely important for me to find them, and this quest was a labor of love. I do hope that this book will inspire other books so we can continue to tell our own stories.

Geoffrey "Geo" Edwards

Geoffrey "Geo" Edwards (he/him/his) is an educator and healing artist whose practice is primarily centered on herbal medicine, art therapy, and gardening. He is the owner of Nu Grain & Pestle LLC, an herb apothecary and plant nursery, and creator of Nu Healing Arts Garden, a teaching garden and incubator for his studio and healing arts practices. In addition to his creative practice, Edwards is a guest lecturer and clinic faculty in the acupuncture program at the Maryland University of Integrative Health. Edwards often facilitates plant walks and workshops on numerous topics ranging from ecology, the five elements, and creative writing, to herb cultivation and art-as-social action. He loves storytelling and building with his wife and sons about all things art, music, genealogy, and food.

I met Geo at the International Herb Symposium and heard him lecture a few times on multiple herbal conference platforms. I had not met many male herbalists of color at that time, especially ones who have the heart that he has. I like to call him "Professor Geo" because he is so dedicated to sharing knowledge. Recently we started the Black Mystery School, a collective of multidisciplinary practitioners teaching our community. Seeing his work in a closer setting, I had to include him in this book because he is unique.

What is the meaning of your name, if you know it, and where are you and your people from?

My name is Geoffrey Eugene Edwards, and I go by Geo. "Geoffrey" means divine peace, also God's peace. Eugene is also my father's name and means well born, noble. I was born and raised in Milwaukee, Wisconsin. My family's maternal side's known story starts in the North Central Hills of Mississippi before Mississippi was a state (late 1700 to early 1800s). My paternal side's story starts in Virginia near the Dismal Swamp area bordering North Carolina. We have no knowledge of the African tribal names or origins, but there is detailed oral history on my maternal side involving deep familial ties with the Chahta (Choctaw) people. Both sides left the central hills and migrated to the Mississippi Delta area in the late 1800s.

Tell us about your work and why it is important to you.

I am a healing artist, emphasis on "healing" and emphasis on "artist." The two are inseparable for me. Art therapy and visual art were the focus of my work before I decided to pursue formal training in East Asian medicine (acupuncture and herbal medicine). However, I come from a family lineage steeped in farming prophecy, visions, ministry with music, laying of hands, and commanding word and spirit. I currently integrate all of this into my healing arts practice and urban gardening work.

Is there a spiritual connection that inspires you in your work?

I only know of one plant that my maternal grandmother Beatrice Fair used, comfrey/knitbone, though our family oral history informs me she was well versed in disappearing into the woods to get herbs. My deep interest and spiritual connection to working topically with plants to heal the wounded is definitely rooted in the stories I know of her using knitbone topically to treat pain and injuries. There also is the spiritual connection of using "blessed oils" and laying of hands on the afflicted that I find as a consistent theme in my family.

What is the importance to you of carrying on the legacy and stories of our people?

Our stories are the bedrock and foundation to understanding any possibility of a future for our people. There are indigenous parts of ourselves that did not go away, were not cultured away, that were not "Westerned" away by colonization but lay dormant in our psyche. These are "underwater" parts of ourselves that can be likened to us having the great civilization of Atlantis within us that were covered by the great flood of European expansionism.

What is it that you would like people to know about your culture, your people, and where you come from?

I am a product of blues and praise breaks, a symphony of deep rivers and great lakes. Black Southern indigenous folks who migrated north and brought quilts, guitars, okra, and mustards with them so we wouldn't forget.

Could you share a few food, herbal medicine, spiritual bath, or skin care recipes that are important to you and your work? Also what do they tell of the story of your culture? What are your favorite plants to work with?

My favorite plants to work are mugwort, okra, mustard seed, castor, fig tree, magnolia tree, peach tree, mulberry tree, goji vine, nettles, and mimosa tree.

Fig, mulberry, magnolia, peach, mustard, and okra were all cultivated by both of my grandfathers, so they have become staples of my practice to maintain the generational continuity.

Mugwort-infused oil is a product that I sell and is also a staple in my acupuncture and bodywork components of my practice. Very simple to make. Start with carrier oil of choice (coconut, olive, almond, castor, etc.). Chop mugwort into smaller pieces to aid infusion. There is a "quick" infusion or "slow" infusion. Feel free to experiment with infusing in the sun. This is not my method, but some people do it this way to capture the solar energy. You can use fresh mugwort if infused with a slow method. For quick infusion with stove/Crock-Pot and low heat, dried mugwort is preferred. Add the herbs to your jar or pot if doing stovetop, enough to cover herbs by an inch or so. Let the mugwort infuse for six to eight hours or overnight. If using the slow method, it really comes down to your preference. Can be one week, two weeks, or a moon cycle, etc. Regardless of method, when the infusion process is complete, strain herbs with fine mesh or cheesecloth several times, then bottle, label, and keep in a cool place out of direct sunlight.

What do you hope that people will learn about where you are from? What would you like to see for the future of Black people in herbalism and/or the healing arts?

I imagine a world where Black herbalists and practitioners of the healing arts are more respected and financially compensated for the time, money, commitment, and sacrifice that goes into studying and becoming stewards of nature, the land, and the various traditions that grow from it. Sometimes I think our people can take for granted all that we offer and the effort it takes to be in the position to offer it.

What does honoring your ancestors mean to you? What practices would you love to share?

I started with and continue to do altar work with my ancestors. Over the past few years, this altar practice has transformed into ancestral gardening, where I cultivate the land and grow the same plants my oral history informs me that my grandfathers grew. We as descendants of indigenous peoples have to regain, reclaim, and decolonize the Western notions of the senses and awaken from deep within ourselves memories of ancestral ways of being and knowing that only exist in our tongues and ears; both as oral histories in our stories and knowledges encoded in the flavors of our foods and herbs.

I would argue that entire worlds of knowing will unfold as we embrace indigenous diets, foods, and flavors. Flavors are the gateway to knowing. There are ancestral memories that will only become accessible when you taste amaranth, yam, and bitter leaf.

What concepts of herbalism do you practice that make your work unique?

My herbal practice is unique in that I have integrated my formal training in East Asian medicine with my gardening practice and the Black indigenous food ways that I have learned from my family's oral history. So there is a significant emphasis on growing and using the foods my ancestors used, however, looking at them from an energetic lens informed by my studies in five element and TCM [traditional Chinese medicine] theories.

Anything else you would love to say about yourself, your work, or teachers that would inspire other herbalists or herbal enthusiasts on their path to connecting to their roots and the plants?

I set out on the path of my herbalist training before digging deep into my genealogy. Although my work is integrated now, I would encourage anyone considering herbalism to do the opposite, as that will help to better inform the type of herb tradition to dive into.

What projects, products, or classes about your medicine and knowledge would you like to share?

Grain and Pestle is the hub for my apothecary and studio art practices. I also plan to integrate my classes and training for adolescents and young adults interested in pursuing herbalism and the healing arts as a path.

Nu Moxa Oil is my signature topical formula for multiple uses related to joint and muscle pain and stiffness.

I have a core selection of classes centered on working with the spoken/written word and sowing seeds, the shared ecology of the body and nature, and the use of moxibustion as a meditative and spiritual practice.

Are there any living herbalists or ancestors that inspire you or whose work you admire?

I admire the work breadth of Dr. Afrika and influence [of] Dr. Sebi. Many facets of my Chinese medical influences are indebted to the work of Dr. Jeffrey. Yuen. My Black Mystery School colleagues (Ayo Ngozi, Karen Culpepper, Lucretia Van Dyke, Karma Mayet, Ikeoma Divine) are my living inspirations and coconspirators. I love Amanda David's work with the People's Medicine School. Other herbalists I have worked extensively with and inspired by the work of [are] Sobande Greer, Stephanie Morningstar, Shabina Lafleur-Gangji, Yuma Bellomee, Khetnu Nefer of Gullah Geechee Herbal Gathering, and Molly Meehan of Wild Ginger herbal center. These are the folks I see myself growing old with in this life work.

Thank you, Geo, for the work you do to carry the legacy of our ancestors!

Contact information:

Instagram: @geo_creativespace
www.nuhealingarts.com

Wilnise Francois

I met Wilnise Francois when we sat on a panel for the herbalist Karen Rose. Before meeting her, I had attended the seminar "Kilti Pye Bwa: A Journey through Earth Stewardship in the Dyaspora Ayisyen," which was taught by Francois in mostly Haitian Creole. I was in tears and blown away in feeling the passion in their own language that they have for the plants, their people, and their ancestors' remedy stories. Francois is a Haitian American licensed nurse and herbalist who worked in the allopathic modality of healing (a system in which medical doctors and other health care professionals treat symptoms and diseases using drugs, surgery, or other medical procedures) for over a decade, working alongside physicians and caretakers alike and facilitating wellness for those of all ages. Her role as an herbalist expanded as she combined her knowledge of both Haitian and Western herbal practices. As a community herbalist, she is working to revolutionize the cultural affinity of our plant friends through our relationships with the earth and stars. Her aim is to integrate the very love our herbs show us and implement that essence into our daily lives, creating a lifestyle of health and wellness.

What is the meaning of your name, if you know it, and where are you and your people from?

The beloved name Wilnise, as emphasized by my father, signifies "sun, moon, and stars." According to Google, the name means "to be devoted."

Tell us about your work and why it is important to you.

My work is a divine theater. The most high, through my ancestors, is the creator/creatress of the scene. The plants serve as the props, and I, the sacred actress, [get] to freely dance in a symphonious garden of love, harmony, death, and resurrection. It is truly the purest way to journey in my destiny. It holds value to me because it's an extension of myself in all essence, and it stands as a reflection of the example I unknowingly wish I had. I wish to be that ancestor that was clear and full to model.

Is there a spiritual connection that inspires you in your work?

In my deepest understanding, all of what I do is spirit. I like to know/believe that spirit is the driving force in all of what I do as an Afrikan being on this planet that speaks heavily in the way we interact and move in the world. Spirit is the balance that keeps all aligned.

My ancestral lineage is the driving force in helping me to recognize that gift from the most high. The way they move in their lives spoke heavily to the trust they have in spirit. That example is the driving force of my sacred work.

What is the importance to you of carrying on the legacy and stories of our people?

For so long I felt this void in my personal lineage because this ingenious information was not preserved. I am the eldest in my family dynamic, so it can also be this stronghold to that role. My calling is the responsibility to preserve and secure this unspoken knowing that we all have. Oral tradition is the framework to our ancestral knowledge. With the access of resources we have now, it is our sole duty to uphold and preserve for generations to come. Spirit has awakened me to the need for action so I followed suit and have been journeying through it ever since.

What is it that you would like people to know about your culture, your people, and where you come from?

Ayiti (Haiti), "flower of highland," is freedom. I would like that resounding truth to be known because it is not only self-evident but a fact that helps to shape the idea of freedom for peoples around the world. That is the spirit and fabric of the *Ayisyen* (Haitian) diaspora. *Ayiti* is love, that deep, sensuous love embellished in the resurrection of spirit and *la nati* (nature). It is through our inner standing of the laws of nature that shapes our character and integrity in the world.

Could you share a few food, herbal medicine, spiritual bath, or skin care recipes that are important to you and your work? Also what do they tell of the story of your culture? What are your favorite plants to work with?

Our aura is the energy that flows through us and around us. It radiates energy from within you and absorbs energy around us. In Ayiti that can sometimes be referred to as our *maji*/essence/our highest and divine self. Activating your *maji* to then nourish the whole body is a practice acknowledged heavily in our culture. Ayisyen herbal baths, or "bains," are baths specific to the alleviation of both physical and spiritual attacks presumed on the body. Whether it be a *lave tet* (washing of the head), a postpartum bain, or a general bain, baths are done to realign the physical and spiritual body into balance.

The bain is done to help clear any stagnation that is found while supplying the body balance. This recipe is a tried-and-true family bain done to foster auric strength at any time.

Bain components are as follows:

* *Fèy assosi* (bitter melon/*Momordica charantia*). This has powerful antiviral properties that can stimulate the immune system and activate the body's natural killer cells to help fight off viruses; it is a powerful energetic cleanser and anti-inflammatory for the skin.

* *Fèy baslik* (holy basil/*Ocimum gratissimum*). Preparations from the whole plant are used in treating sunstroke (*dekonboze*), headache (*tèt fe mal*), and influenza (*lafyèv*). The anti-inflammatory, antibacterial, antiseptic properties are why it is most used topically.

* *Pèsi* (parsley/*Petroselinum crispum*). This is long known for its skin-refreshing and toning properties; it has been used for years for its ability to clean and soothe skin. Parsley is often used in baths to help with bruising since it soothes inflammation.

* *Sel*: Salt to purify

FAMILY BATH

This may be done beforehand and preserved over time to be used when called. To personalize the bath, adding essential oils like lemongrass or citrus to the mixture to amplify set intentions is also helpful.

1 cup fresh or dried
bitter melon vine

1 cup fresh or dried holy basil

½ cup fresh or dried parsley

1 teaspoon salt

1. Start by mixing the dry ingredients together in the large bowl. Add the mixture to the jars and label them with their ingredients and the date crafted. Add a couple of tablespoons to each bath whenever you feel called.

2. You can do this bath at any time. The bath is to cleanse your energy and your spirit.

What do you hope that people will learn about where you are from? What would you like to see for the future of Black people in herbalism and/or the healing arts?

I feel we are in the midst of the most revolutionary era we have seen as a people.

All very familiar yet new, and for me that helps to bring an awareness of just how far we as a people have to go. At our best we shine and excel in all of it. The reclamation and remembering echoing our communities allows for us to be at ease for the new world that we were all consciously creating together. My greatest knowing is that we stay the course and continue to foster the framework of community for our loved ones. We are here blooming, creating, birthing our new world and it is an honor to be in the midst of it.

What does honoring your ancestors mean to you? What practices would you love to share?

Honoring ancestors to me is waking each day and taking my first breath. I believe the ancestors reveal in my lived experience and I feel each waking step is an ode and honor to them. The way I honor my ancestors is holding myself accountable to the divine of expression of my nature while carving specific time that helps to exonerate their work and dreams.

What concepts of herbalism do you practice that make your work unique?

My work with plants is deeply rooted in the awakening of spirit communication. I feel the inclination and nudge from the plants calls for this deep dive into the sublime that allows for full expression of creativity to emerge. Because the conversation is so personal, any way I am with the plants, be it forging, tending, or using in medicine, makes it all specific to my personal expression in the world. There's a focus layered in not only what I may receive from our interaction but what message the plants may want to deliver.

Is there any advice to an aspiring herbalist?

I believe there's an herbalist tucked in every being on this planet and whenever I get to witness anyone sitting in that role, sharing in whatever way, inspires me. It really helps to amplify the work we all feel so called to reclaim.

Contact information:

Instagram: @wellfedapothecary and @wilnise (Her pages are pure plant inspiration!)
www.wellfedapothecary.com

Olatokunboh "Ola" Obasi

There is so much I can say about Olatokunboh "Ola" Obasi; she inspires me so much, but I will let her words tell you.

Obasi is the owner of Omaroti, an apothecary and wellness space in Mayagüez, Puerto Rico. Obasi has been working in the wellness field for over fifteen years. She is a yoga and dance instructor, clinical herbalist, nutritionist, and birth doula. Committed to community holistic health, social justice, and education, she works heavily in community service and African traditional medicine. She coordinates Herbalists without Borders International on the island and provides devotional service to people in need with her free clinics every Thursday.

A guest presenter and teacher in many conferences, she integrates traditional knowledge of herbs with her Western education. She received her masters of science from the Maryland University of Integrative Health. Obasi is also a mother of three young adults. She continues to learn from her children through challenge and tribulation as she shares her journey of life with them and the human family. She works with clients clinically in private sessions to provide wellness and holistic health through herbal medicines.

What is the meaning of your name, if you know it, and where are you and your people from?

My name is Olatokunboh Obasi. It is a Yoruba name that literally means honor the one born from the water (ocean) and is given to children who are born abroad, not in Nigeria. My father is Nigerian, my mother Kenyan and Ethiopian. But I was conceived in Kenya, born in the US while my mother was a student and returned to Kenya with her four years later after her studies, thus my name.

Tell us about your work and why it is important to you.

My work is very important to me because it's a continuation of a family legacy. My work began as a child; I grew up mostly all over East Africa and spent a lot of time in my maternal village with my grandparents. There I learned to respect nature and the many realms of life. This laid a foundation for my work in herbalism and healing arts. As a clinical herbalist and nutritionist, I also support people's health choices and guide them to wellness. I truly enjoy seeing people well, motivated to be well and moving into a direction of empowerment.

Is there a spiritual connection that inspires you in your work or people that you have and would love to share?

I am an *Iyaawonifa,* a priestess in the *Ifá* tradition. I am also a Tekina in the Taino tradition. These very unique and humbling paths pave the foundation for my spirit ways. I and my children received the honor of adaptation in the Taino community over the course of ten years. Since both of these converge in an indigenous sense, my spiritual connection comes from an indigenous root. I have had many teachers along the way (as a citizen of the planet). My parents were diplomats, so I had the honor to travel often, especially around Africa. I have been taught by a Zulu medicine man and woman in South Africa, a Tswana medicine man when my parents lived in the Kalahari area of Botswana. I have teachers from my village and Ile Ife, Nigeria, where my teacher *(oluwo)* lives. My most important teachers have been my great-uncle, who was my first herb teacher, named Olwaya, and my current Taino mother, named Kukuya. Divine interventions along the path of life have brought me a magical and spiritual connection that inspires and informs all facets of my life.

What is the importance to you of carrying on the legacy and stories of our people?

Legacy is what I live for. We are all guaranteed to die, so death is imminent for all of us. Afro and Afro indigenous stories are very important to ensure inheritance and guidance for the future generations along the way of life. Legacy and story are purposefully part of my practice. They also guarantee eternal life. In essence our stories are immortal. And that is the importance of carrying on the legacy of our people!

Could you share a few food, herbal medicine, spiritual bath, or skin care recipes that are important to you and your work? Also what do they tell of the story of your culture? What are your favorite plants to work with?

Since living on the island of *Borinquén*[34] for more than five years, my practice has shifted from what it was in the United States to becoming more earth connected. I think more like plants. I truly understand more now than ever the importance of adapting and connecting with the environment we live in. The plants tell the stories and here they tell of the cultures that have influenced the accepted culture. Like most places, it's a melting pot. In Kenya, for instance, a lot of our herbs and practices are common to the Indus Valley and the Middle East. In Borinquén, the plants that are used by local country folks are mostly Taino and African in origin and practice. Many of the African plants are from specific areas of Africa.

For example, oregano brujo, *Plectranthus amboinicus*, is directly connected to the Congo Bantu people, who were brought here enslaved from central East Africa. Being that this is a plant that

---

34 Puerto Ricans often call the island Borinquén, a derivation of Borikén, its indigenous Taíno name, which means "Land of the Valiant Lord." See Paul Allatson, *Key Terms in Latino/a Cultural and Literary Studies* (Malden, MA: Blackwell Publishing, 2007), 47.

is semisucculent and can endure vibrancy for months, it also is simple to propagate—just plant the leaf and stem into the soil; it grows easily and is hard to kill. This has to be one of my most favorite plants here. I see the story of farmers, diviners, and mothers carrying this plant in their hair, in their armpits, or even in their buttocks, to carry familiar medicine to the unknown lands that they were forced to go. Now we have evidence of this green print. My mother is part Congo Bantu, and in her mother tongue, the plant would be called Shilauha, in some other areas it may be called okita or akita. I like to add this plant to a pot of beans or stews. I use this same plant for spiritual baths for protection and vitality as well as cleaning the house with it. And I like it as an ingredient in herbal oils and liniments as an anti-inflammatory, antispasmodic, antiallergic, and antibacterial.

What would you like to see for the future of Black people in herbalism and/or the healing arts?

We are everywhere we are called to be. People who are attracted to my work and practice are meant to walk with me. In the big picture, Black people should be more present in all forums of herbalism. Speaking of our unique relationships and connections with our medicine, we should be honored for our knowledge that has supported all other people on this planet as well. And we should work together more often and form our own herbalism, healing art institution(s). I would like to see us collaborate more.

What concepts of herbalism do you practice that make your work unique?

I practice a lot of free community service and involve both my spiritual and academic background in my practice. This helps to guide our sessions effortlessly with a protocol that is both spiritually based herbs and clinically based herbs. Many times they overlap since they're not really separate. In a nutshell, this practice of herbalism feeds our souls because to me it is an offering that generates abundance for all involved.

What projects or classes do you offer?

I have a school that keeps me very busy, Well of Indigenous Wisdom School. I offer new classes three to four times a year. I also enjoy guest teaching at other schools and get especially excited when I am invited to POC (people of color) herb schools, etc. I continue to do service work in Borinquén and teach as well as provide clinical service on the island as long as my ancestors want me here.

Contact information:

Instagram: @omarotiwellofindigenouswisdom
www.wellofindigenouswisdom.com

Khetnu Nefer

I am so inspired my Khetnu Nefer's love of her people. The Gullah Geechee people are such an important part of our history. Her conference gives a rare opportunity for people of color to gather and learn from each other in a safe environment dedicated to our stories. Khetnu Nefer (LaDawn Frasier) is a Gullah Geechee holistic health practitioner from John's Island, South Carolina, who is a passionate womb warrior and women's health advocate. An Army veteran, uterine cancer survivor, and licensed massage therapist of seventeen years, Nefer fuses modalities to assist women on their path to well-being. She is a self-published author, professional African dancer, Egyptian yoga instructor, herbalist, certified birth doula, certified kukuwa African dance instructor, and former massage professor.

As a graduate of the American College of Healthcare Sciences in Portland, Oregon, Nefer established her mobile holistic wellness company A Soulful Touch Wellness, where she provides workshops, products, and services. Nefer is also the founder of the Gullah Geechee Herbal Gathering, an up-and-coming herbal conference for Black and indigenous herbalists in South Carolina. Nefer is a proud member of Kappa Epsilon Psi Military Sorority, the Collective Health Initiative, and WoVeN (Women's Veteran Network).

What is the meaning of your name, if you know it, and where are you and your people from?

My birth name is LaDawn Frasier, but most people know me professionally as my Spiritual name Khetnu Nefer, which is ancient Egyptian for "as I serve God, I achieve success." I am from a coastal sea island in South Carolina within the Gullah Geechee heritage corridor called Johns Island, South Carolina. My people are mostly Gullah Geechee from South Carolina, but I also have French and Haitian ancestry on my father's side.

Tell us about your work and why it is important to you.

My work primarily revolves around women's health, most specifically womb health. I started out as a massage therapist and evolved into an herbalist, holistic health coach, yoga instructor, full spectrum doula, and African dance instructor. I ventured into womb health after my own uterine cancer scare. I used various herbs and holistic health modalities to overcome that naturally and I wanted to be not only an inspiration but a source of holistic health solutions for other women as well.

Most recently, I founded an annual herbal conference for Black and indigenous herbalists called the Gullah Geechee Herbal Gathering. This is a sacred place for Black herbalists, healers, body workers, birth workers, farmers, and the community to converge, learn, network, and support one another. Educating and assisting those who look like me is very important to me and I make it a point to support my community and my heritage in that way.

Is there a spiritual connection that inspires you in your work?

Being a Gullah Geechee country girl who grew up on a coastal sea island, there has always been a strong connection to nature for me. That connection definitely inspires my work. Nature has its own means of balance. I believe that spirituality is the evidence of the experience of one's own nature deep within themselves and how it correlates with others and our environment.

What is the importance to you of carrying on the legacy and stories of our people?

It is important for me to carry on the legacy and stories of my people because now is our time for reclamation and preservation. The legacy and traditions of the Gullah Geechee people have been commodified for so long by people who don't look like us for so long and I believe that it's time for us to amplify and curate our own contributions. Through the Gullah Geechee Herbal Gathering, I have learned how vitally important this is for our culture, especially for those who have felt far removed from the culture.

What is it that you would like people to know about your culture, your people, and where you came from?

The Gullah Geechee people are an amazing legacy of the determination, resilience, ingenuity, and pride of those enslaved individuals that were unwillingly brought to America from West Africa. We are the direct descendants of those people and we have beautifully preserved a lot of their traditions. Gullah Geechee people have lived off the land for centuries, and our connection to our West African roots resembles that. It is important for people to know that Gullah Geechee people are still here and making a concerted effort to not only preserve our heritage, but we're curating our history and forging new paths with our heritage intact.

What are your favorite plants to work with?

Some of my favorite plants to work with are nettle, life everlasting (a Gullah Geechee staple), mullein, red raspberry leaf, motherwort, ashwagandha, and lemon balm. My grandfather used to make an effective cold remedy infusion with Rock and Rye, rock candy, life everlasting, and lemon. I remember getting this as a child and how effective it was in busting up colds and the flu. They would serve it hot as a tea, then wrap you up in blankets. You would sweat through the night and when you woke up in the morning, you would feel so much better. I don't know the exact measurements, but it is definitely one of my favorite herbal memories.

What do you hope that people will learn about where you are from? What would you like to see for the future of Black people in herbalism and/or the healing arts?

I would like to see more involvement and more acknowledgment of our contributions and works for the future of Black people in herbalism and the healing arts. I would like for us to continue to build our own herbal academies and conferences. We also need to produce more publications, training, and opportunities for each other. There is such a wealth of knowledge and wisdom that I believe that has been truly untapped and often overlooked that can help to elevate those in these industries. I would love to see less competition and gatekeeping. Unity and collective economics are vital for us to elevate and prosper as a community.

What does honoring your ancestors mean to you? What practices would you love to share?

Honoring my ancestors is not only an opportunity to acknowledge their presence in my life, but it's also a tremendous source of healing, empowerment, and nourishment for my life. One of my favorite practices to honor them is visiting their grave sites and leaving offerings of either one of their favorite things or some beautiful flowers. I also like to dedicate acts of service and other positive works in my life and business in their honor. Another thing is having an ancestral altar; this serves as a special meeting place to communicate and pay homage to my ancestors. This is a consecrated place and so necessary in my life.

Anything else you would love to say about yourself, your work, or teachers that would inspire other herbalists or herbal enthusiasts on their path to connecting to their roots and the plants?

My work is definitely community focused and orientated. I pride myself for being of service to my community and giving back to them through various aspects of my business to include free community clinics, the Gullah Geechee Herbal Gathering, and my massage therapy. I would definitely say my work is an homage to the Black and indigenous herbalists and healers that came before me and to my current contemporaries. I am inspired by the works and examples of amazing herbalists like you, Lucretia, Yuma "Docta Yew" Bellomee, Ayo Ngozi Drayton, Geo Edwards, Khet Waas Hutip, HerbSistah Eshe Faizah, Dr. Sebi, Dr. Llaila Afrika, and the likes. My maternal grandmother Victoria Thelma Murray was my first herbal teacher, and I am grateful for her example and her wisdom.

What projects, products, or classes are you working on to share your medicine and knowledge with people?

The Gullah Geechee Herbal Gathering is my biggest and most notable project. With it I can align and collaborate with other Black and indigenous herbalists who embody what I want to convey to the community through my works. It is my pride and joy and my ancestral assignment. I teach online workshops as well on various topics from womb health, massage therapy, essential oils, and other health and wellness topics. My "The Fourteen Day Self-Love Experience" course has been very well received by the attendees, and I am working on a corresponding course for my book *28 Days to a Soulful Life*.

Contact information:

Instagram: @asoulfultouchwellness
www.asoulfultouch.net

To learn more about the Gullah Geechee Herbal Gathering, visit:

Instagram: @gullahgeecheeherbs
www.gullahgeecheeherbalgathering.com

Ayodele Ngozi

Ayodele Ngozi is such a force in the herbalist community. Her class was what inspired me to begin the quest of writing this book. Ngozi is a community herbalist, educator, and artist. Trained as a clinician, Ngozi is an instructor at community-based herbal schools and conferences, is a cofounder of the Black Mystery School, and in 2020 created the Planting Reparations Project, a reparations-based, mutual aid initiative that redistributes plants and healing resources to Black people. Ngozi is committed to learning from ancestral tradition, documenting herbal and cultural practices, and serving the community.

What is the meaning of your name, if you know it, and where are you and your people from?

I chose my name, Ayodele Ngozi, when I turned twenty-one. Both of these names are from what we now call Nigeria; Ayodele means "joy has come home" in the Yoruba language, and "Ngozi" means "blessing" in Igbo. Many years later, I learned that my grandmothers' lineages are Yoruba and Igbo! I grew up in Massachusetts, but my family's near roots are in the South—Virginia and South Carolina.

Tell us about your work and why it is important to you.

I am a community herbalist, educator, and visual artist. My work is important to me on so many levels. On a community level, practicing as an herbalist and teaching others reminds me of that saying about teaching a person to fish—whether I'm with a client or in a classroom, the most important thing to me is passing along information and skills to help people be more self-sufficient and confident in tending their own wellness.

On an individual level, working with plants and creating art have both been integral in my personal healing. One thing I love about both is that there is simply no end to the journey of learning and practice.

Is there a spiritual connection that inspires you in your work?

I grew up in the country, and as a child it was nature—the forests and mountains and rivers—that seemed most like God to me. I think I inherited that perspective from generations of ancestors who lived on the land. My great-great-grandparents were herbalists who served their community in and around Locust Dale, Virginia, in the 1800s and very early 1900s, and my spiritual connection to them, and some of the ancestors that came before them, is very strong.

Could you share a few food, herbal medicine, spiritual bath, or skin care recipes that are important to you and your work? Also what do they tell of the story of your culture? What are your favorite plants to work with?

Two herbs that I always associate with my family are dandelion and calamus. I'm a descendant of Africans, who were enslaved in the US, and the fact that these herbs were so important to my ancestors says a lot about the culture of this country and how herbal knowledge was shared, borrowed, and adapted. For example, I like to imagine that my grandmother's legendary dandelion wine, perfected in Virginia, is a way that her folks adapted to the absence of palm wine. It's so hard to name favorite plants when there are so many to choose from, but stinging nettles, ginger, shatavari, Reishi, rose, and marshmallow are way up on my list. And indigo, always indigo.

What do you hope that people will learn about where you are from? What would you like to see for the future of Black people in herbalism and/or the healing arts?

I would most love for more Black healers to be "unbought and unbossed," to quote Shirley Chisholm,[35] and exercise our agency within our respective fields. To me, this means creating schools and training opportunities, writing and publishing books and journals, hosting more conferences and retreats. This isn't about solely operating in BIPOC-only or Black-only spaces but knowing that we can show up in our fullness and authority wherever we are.

---

35 Shirley Chisholm was the first Black woman elected to the United States Congress and represented New York's 12th congressional district for seven terms from 1969 to 1983. In 1972, she became the first Black candidate to seek a major party's nomination for president of the United States. National Archives, African American Heritage, "Shirley Chisholm," https://www.archives.gov/research/african-americans/individuals/shirley-chisholm.

What does honoring your ancestors mean to you? What practices would you love to share?

For me, honoring my ancestors means being mindful about moving through my life in a way that ensures that their efforts, traumas, and sacrifices were not in vain. It means cultivating joy and liberation and pleasure and discipline.

I've maintained a vibrant daily devotional practice at my ancestral altar for the last twenty years. I offer them light, water, food, songs, flowers, etc., but the most important offering is my presence, time, and energy and love. I am so clear that my ancestors have my back, front, and sides, and I'm grateful for that.

Anything else you would love to say about yourself, your work, or teachers that would inspire other herbalists or herbal enthusiasts on their path to connecting to their roots and the plants?

The plants themselves are the greatest teachers! When we can focus and be with them, to observe how they grow, how they taste and smell and feel and land in our bodies, we can learn so much. I've received this teaching in different forms from many folks, but one of my favorites is George Washington Carver.[36]

It's important to remember too that we are all descended from herbalists and healers somewhere in our lineages (we wouldn't be here if we weren't), and when we choose this walk we're just tapping back into something that has been in us from the beginning.

---

36 George Washington Carver was a formerly enslaved Black American agricultural chemist, agronomist, and experimenter whose development of new products derived from peanuts (groundnuts), sweet potatoes, and soybeans helped revolutionize the agricultural economy of the South. "George Washington Carver," Brittanica.com, https://www.britannica.com /biography/George-Washington-Carver.

AFRICAN AMERICAN HERBALISM

What projects, products, or classes are you working on to share your medicine and knowledge with people?

I am always teaching, writing, and making medicine. But what I am most excited about these days is my work with Black Mystery School—we are growing a beautiful community that connects us to our various healing traditions and to one another.

Contact information:

Instagram: @ayo.herbalist
www.thecreativeroot.net
www.blackmysteryschool.org

APPENDIX A:
MAJOR ORISHAS

ORISHA	ATTRIBUTES
Obatala	❁ Creator of human bodies ❁ Elder of the orishas ❁ Represents the crown chakra and brings peace and balance
Elegba	❁ Messenger between two worlds, of the humans and the divine ❁ Keeper of the crossroads and opens the way for new beginnings ❁ Enhances the power of plants and all things by opening up the pathways of communication
Ogun	❁ Orisha of iron and represents the warrior in ourselves; called on for protection ❁ Path maker with his tools of iron ❁ Clearer of paths, specifically blockages in or interruption of the flow energy in the body
Yemoja	❁ Mother of waters (both rivers and saltwater), symbolized by the amniotic fluid in the womb of the pregnant woman ❁ Protective energy of the feminine

ORISHA	ATTRIBUTES
Oshun	✿ Sweetness, sensuality, beauty, and gracefulness ✿ Symbolizes self-clarity and flowing abundance, has power to heal with fresh water; the embodiment of the female essence ✿ Receives prayers from women for fertility and the alleviation of female disorders ✿ Fond of babies; her help is sought if a baby becomes ill ✿ Known for her love of sweet things like honey ✿ Known as the freshwater goddess (lakes and rivers)
Shango	✿ Characteristics include being royal, a protector, masculine beauty, fire, and lightning ✿ Some say he has the ability to transform a base substance into a more valuable one ✿ Teaches us to pull our power down from the heavens
Oya	✿ Female warrior, deity of death and guardian of the cemetery; helps those cross over to the spirit world after dying ✿ Represented by the wind or "the winds of change"
Osain	✿ Deity of healing ✿ Has the knowledge of all the plants for offerings and medicinal purposes ✿ Ruler of the forest, who is revered by the hunters

Source: Janet Evans, *Spirit of the Orisha*, trans. Omoba Adewale Adenle (New Orleans, LA: Sula Spirit LLC, 2014).

APPENDIX B: ANCESTOR QUESTIONNAIRE

Interview an elder or research your own ancestral roots:

Do you know where your ancestors come from?

What plants medicines did they use, and how did they use them?

Have you or anyone in your immediate family used plant medicine? What are some favorites?

_____

_____

_____

_____

_____

_____

_____

What family medicinal recipes have been passed down?

_____

_____

_____

_____

_____

_____

_____

REFERENCES

"A Brief History of Jim Crow." Constitutional Rights Foundation. https://www.crf-usa.org/black-history-month/a-brief-history-of-jim-crow.

Allatson, Paul. *Key Terms in Latino/a Cultural and Literary Studies*. Malden, MA: Blackwell Publishing, 2007.

Ames, Hana. "What Are the Benefits of Shea Butter?" *Medical News Today*. April 21, 2021. https://www.medicalnewstoday.com/articles/shea-butter-benefits#types.

Blanton, Wyndham Bolling. *Medicine in Virginia in the 18th Century*. University of Michigan: Garrett & Massie, 1931.

Boutlern Carmen, dir. *The Pyramid Code*. Episode 1, "The Band of Peace." Aired 2009.

Cavender, Anthony. *Folk Medicine in Southern Appalachia*. Chapel Hill: University of North Carolina Press, 2003.

Easley, Thomas and Steven Horne. *The Modern Herbal Dispensatory: A Medicine Making Guide*. Berkeley, CA: North Atlantic Books, 2016.

"Ebers Papyrus," in Brittanica.com, https://www.britannica.com/topic/Ebers-papyrus.

"Edwin Smith Papyrus," in Brittanica.com, https://www.britannica.com/topic/Edwin-Smith-papyrus.

"The European Market Potential for Shea Butter." *CBI.edu*. Last updated February 10, 2021. https://www.cbi.eu/market-information/natural-ingredients-cosmetics/shea-butter/market-potential.

Evans, Janet. *Spirit of the Orisha*. Translated by Omoba Adewale Adenle. New Orleans, LA: Sula Spirit LLC, 2014.

"Herbal Medicine FAQs." *American Herbalists Guild*. https://www.americanherbalistsguild.com/herbal-medicine-fundamentals.

Kandola, Aaron. "Benefits of Castor Oil for the Face and Skin." *Medical News Today*. June 28, 2018. https://www.medicalnewstoday.com/articles/319844.

Karade, Baba Ifa, *The Handbook of Yoruba Religious Concepts*. Newburyport, MA: Weiser Books, 1994.

Lee, Michele. *Working the Roots: Over 400 Years of African American Healing*. Oakland, CA: Wadastick Publishers, 2014.

Logan, Annie Lee. Mot*herwit: An Alabama Midwife's Story*. San Francisco, CA: Untreed Reads, 2013.

National Archives, African American Heritage, "Shirley Chisholm." https:// www.archives.gov/research/african-americans/individuals/shirley -chisholm.

Patton, Darryl. *Mountain Medicine: The Herbal Remedies of Tommie Bass*. Mount Vernon, VA: Little River Press, 2017.

Pearson, Calvin. *The History and Legacy of the 1619 Enslaved African Landing*. Project 1619 Inc, 2021.

Penniman, Leah. *Farming While Black: Soul Fire Farm's Practical Guide to Liberation on the Land*. Hartford, VT: Chelsea Green Publishing, 2018.

Pilgrim, David. "What Was Jim Crow." Ferris State University. https://www .ferris.edu/HTMLS/news/jimcrow/what.htm.

Savitt, Todd L. *Medicine and Slavery: The Diseases and Health Care of Blacks in Antebellum Virginia*. Urbana, IL: University of Illinois Press, 1978.

Sawandi, Tariq "Yorubic Medicine: The Art of Divine Herbology." Accessed February 9, 2022. https://planetherbs.com/research-center/theory -articles/yorubic-medicine-the-art-of-divine-herbology.

Smallwood, Stephanie E. *Saltwater Slavery: A Middle Passage from Africa to American Diaspora*. Cambridge, MA: Harvard University Press, 2008.

Swannanoa Valley Museum. "Catching Babies: Midwife Mary Stepp Burnette Hayden." Swannanoa Valley Museum & History Center. April 23, 2018. https://www.history.swannanoavalleymuseum.org/catching-babies -midwife-mary-stepp-burnette-hayden.

Williams, Paige. "Herbalist, 94, Lets Nature Heal." *Tulsa World*. Last updated February 25, 2019. https://tulsaworld.com/archive/herbalist-94-lets -nature-heal/article_3b0e06d1-4af9-5567-93ee-bc4b50d5867f.html.

ACKNOWLEDGMENTS

To all the teachers who guided me on this journey to be healed and embraced my role as a healer: a deep bow of gratitude to you!

This work is to honor my family for their knowledge of working with the earth. This knowledge that lies deep in my bones. I'm thankful for the support of my mother and sister during this process, as well as for my brother for being my first herbal "client" when we were children.

This is for my tribe family—Gina, Ikeoma, Sula, and Joy—your amazing sisterhood helped me see my light when I couldn't. Thank you also to my love for cheering me on every day writing this. Y'all ROCK! I have so much gratitude for you all!

To dear beloved Valarie Boyd, who told me I too could be a writer and inspired me and others to tell the stories. Thank you! You are truly missed!

Thank you to my chosen family, friends, students, and colleagues for your sweet messages of encouragement; much gratitude for telling the stories of why this work matters. I have truly appreciated every one of them.

Thank you to Auntie's favorite mermaid and nature element child Camdyn; you help keep my soul at play. May this book help you know you can do anything!

I hope this work makes those who feel alone on their journey know that they are seen and their stories matter.

ABOUT THE AUTHOR

With a journey that began when she was a little girl mixing herbs, mud, and roots on her grandparents' farm, Lucretia VanDyke has had a life-long connection to the plants. She has been in the wellness industry for over twenty-five years. Her quest for knowledge and storytelling has led her all over the world to learn about remedies, traditions, and ceremonies from indigenous healers.

One of the foremost experts on Southern folk healing arts, Lucretia integrates rituals, plant spirit meditation, holistic food/herbal medicine, and ancestor reverence into people's practices.

Lucretia has worked and trained with many internationally known spa and skin care companies. She is a holistic educator, speaker, herbalist, sacred sexologist, ceremonialist, spiritual coach, intuitive energy practitioner, diviner, author, and world traveler. Lucretia brings her vivacious spirit and her message of ancestral connection in herbal practices to inspire others to embrace their unique relationship with the plants.

Teaching herbal classes, cooking, storytelling, and foraging in the woods learning native medicine charges her soul.